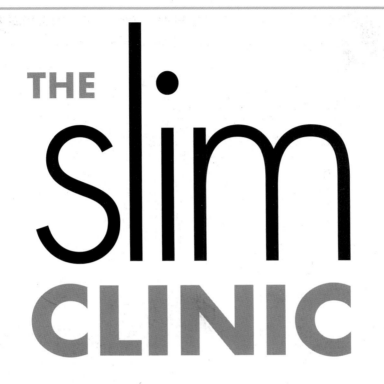

THE slim CLINIC

Hospital-approved programmes that **guarantee** to change
your attitude to food and dieting **permanently**

Dr Marjon Monfared

CARROLL & BROWN PUBLISHERS LIMITED

To my mother, Mary, whose strength and kindness has been my support and inspiration

First published in 2005 in the United Kingdom by

Carroll & Brown Publishers Limited
20 Lonsdale Road
London NW6 6RD

Project editor Ian Wood
Designer Laura De Grasse

A CIP catalogue record for this book is available from the British Library.

ISBN 1-904760-06-6

10 9 8 7 6 5 4 3 2 1

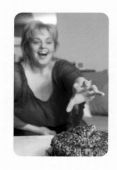

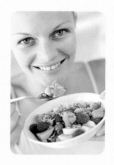

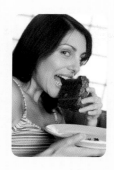

Reproduced by Colourscan, Singapore
Printed and bound in Italy by LEGO

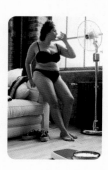

MIDLOTHIAN LIBRARY SERVICE

Please return/renew this item by the last date shown.
To renew please give your borrower number.
Renewal may be made in person, online,
by post, email or phone.

MD.2

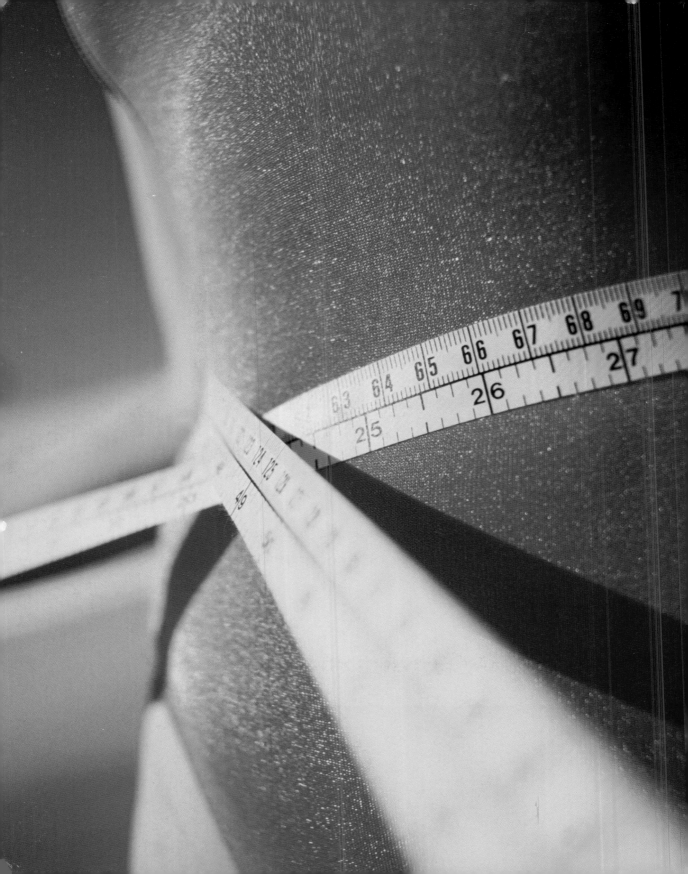

CONTENTS

1 FOOD, ENERGY AND WEIGHT

3 CAUSES OF OVEREATING

2 APPETITE AND DIGESTION

4 HOW TO CONTROL YOUR WEIGHT

INTRODUCTION

All over the Western world, ever-increasing numbers of people are falling prey to what the World Health Organization defines as 'A disease state in which excess fat has accumulated to an extent that health may be adversely affected'. This condition – obesity – now affects about 21 percent of men and 24 percent of women the United Kingdom, and these percentages are rising. In the United States, the percentage of men who are obese has risen from 22 percent in 1994 to 33 percent today, and that of women from 31 percent to 40 percent. What is causing this seemingly unstoppable rise?

Government agencies and the media are constantly telling us that we need to lose weight, and as a result we are spending more than ever on weight-loss products and services, yet the number of people struggling to lose weight is still rising. So where are we going wrong? Why do so many of us find it so hard to lose weight and to keep it off? We have conquered most of the adversities that the natural world has thrown at us, and yet we never imagined that one of the greatest threats to our survival could be too much food. So why and how did this happen?

GENETICS AND ENVIRONMENT

The main problem appears to lie in a basic mismatch between our inherent genetic tendencies and our environment in the West today. Food provides the energy that sustains life at its basic level and, unlike us, our ancestors lived in an environment in which food supply was not guaranteed. The amount of food that previous generations used to eat was limited by its availability, and the biggest threat to their survival was famine. Only those humans who were able to eat more than they needed when food was available, and store it as body fat for when it was scarce, would have survived. In fact, humans who had difficulty gaining weight, and whose metabolisms were less efficient at saving calories, would have been at a distinct disadvantage.

It is a similar story with physical activity. Our ancestors were much more active than we are, out of need and not necessarily desire. It was the drive to survive that forced our predecessors into activity, to find food and to run from danger, and those who were not active were more likely to perish.

Within the past century, and particularly in the past forty years, our lives in the West have been transformed beyond recognition. Famine is by far the least threat to our survival and we no longer have to be active. Food is plentiful and readily available. It is also highly palatable and able to bypass many of the control systems that naturally regulate our food intake. So as well as our genes, our environment – which used to be a barrier to weight gain – now also actively encourages it. Our environment has therefore been described as 'obesogenic'. Our bodies have basically not had enough time to adapt to this new environment. We are driven by an innate desire to eat and have not evolved the physiological or psychological ability to eat less, or to exercise more, simply by applying willpower.

If you take individuals who are hard-wired with the tendency to overeat and put on weight, and put them in an environment that promotes the consumption of high-calorie foods and drinks, but at the same time provides motorized transport and sedentary occupations, then weight gain is the natural outcome. In fact, the surprising thing is that the number of people who are overweight is not actually higher.

PSYCHOLOGICAL ISSUES

It is not just eating too much and exercising too little, however, that can lead to weight gain. Some of us have developed a damaging emotional relationship with certain foods so we eat for the wrong reasons, while others eat at the wrong times and in the wrong ways because of personal or work circumstances and commitments. Some people have simply fallen into bad patterns of eating, out of habit rather than choice. More often than not, a combination of these factors has conditioned us to rely on external cues rather than our own internal appetite-control mechanisms to tell us when and how much to eat. Relying on these external cues is, on the whole, an inefficient way of regulating our food intake.

As a result, many of us in the West now struggle against our own genetic tendencies and our environment in a constant battle to lose weight. This is a battle that is all too often lost as we endlessly search for and try out different ways of shedding weight. The lure of the latest fad diet, exercise machine or dietary supplement means that we end up spending collective millions on products that ultimately disappoint, leaving us further disillusioned by what we believe, mistakenly, to be our own weakness and failure. In addition, the inherently dysfunctional cult of dieting encourages us to go through cycles of weight loss and weight gain. This is not only psychologically damaging and counterproductive but also, by making our bodies more efficient at storing fat, encourages weight gain in the long run.

TIME FOR CHANGE

This book aims to help you find the right strategy to manage your weight over your lifetime, to optimize your health and increase your chances of a long and rewarding life. Part of that strategy has to include a basic understanding of the mechanisms that influence your weight and appetite. You also need to know how weight changes in themselves can affect these mechanisms, and develop an awareness of the external and social cues that can manipulate your dietary choices, eating behaviour and activity levels.

Gaining this knowledge will help you to identify the root causes of your weight gain or your inability to lose weight. It will also form the foundation on which you can build the dietary and lifestyle modifications that will help you achieve and maintain long-term weight loss.

The following are the most common patterns of lifestyle and eating behaviours that often lead to weight gain or prevent weight loss. I have given a very basic outline of the problem, the issues that each raises, and possible 'cures' that we will expand upon in later chapters. These types of behaviour do not necessarily present in isolation: you can be a grazing chocoholic, for example, and live an inactive life on top of that.

1 DISORDERED EATING

This is the person who tends to skip breakfast and eats little throughout the day, but by the end of the day is quite hungry, and on returning home is unable to control his or her appetite and overeats, often right up until bed. He or she may also have had to shop for food after work, at which time they may have been more tempted to buy unhealthy foods to eat later. The pattern is feast and famine, which tends to make the body more efficient at storing fat. This type of eating behaviour is also seen in busy working mums and shift workers. The person is trying to override their natural hunger cues and so the answer here is to re-establish eating in response to hunger/satiety cues and to balance out calorie intake throughout the day.

2 GRAZING

This pattern of continuous eating throughout the day (and evening) is often seen amongst stay-at-home mums, those who work from home, are retired, or work in the catering industry. These people tend not to have proper sit-down meals, but pick on small snacks throughout the day – constant feasting. It is very hard to keep track of the amount of food being consumed in one day when you snack in this way and it is also harder for the body to regulate food intake physiologically because it does not experience hunger/satiety cues that correlate with meal times. People often end up taking in many more calories than they realize. The answer is to set specific time for eating and retuning to hunger/satiety cues.

3 PASSIVE OVERCONSUMPTION

This results from a lack of awareness of the nutritional and calorie content of foods being consumed on a regular basis. It occurs most commonly when food is not prepared and cooked at home and is one of the major causes of weight gain among the general population in recent times. Busy lifestyles mean that many now eat out in restaurants or rely on takeaways and convenience ready-made meals and snacks for their food. These are often calorie-dense, high in hidden fats and sugars with little fibre, so that although there is no volitional intent on the part of the consumer to overeat, it is possible to take in a large number of calories in a short space of time before feeling full. The answer is to develop a greater awareness of nutrition and try to reduce reliance on food retailers.

4 INSATIABLE APPETITE

This person complains of feeling hungry all the time. People with an
insatiable appetite can't stop eating and feel out of control. This is
particularly common in people whose diets are high in carbohydrates,
especially of foods made with refined carbohydrates such as white bread
and sugar. Consumption of these foods appears to trigger their appetite and
so they overeat. The answer is to eat a more balanced diet to help control
appetite by increasing the amount of protein and/or healthy fats and
switching to carbohydrates with a higher fibre content and a lower
glycaemic index.

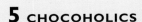

5 CHOCOHOLICS

Snacking in between meals on high calorie, sugary foods and drinks can add
substantially to daily calorie intake and is a major hurdle to weight loss. A
craving for such foods, especially chocolate, is very common among women, and particularly at
certain times in their monthly cycles. Such individuals may have an otherwise healthy diet and
feel sated by eating regular portions at meal times but give in to cravings for fatty, sugary snacks
in between. The answer here is to help curb cravings by consuming a diet aimed at keeping
blood sugar levels stable and to employ techniques that aim to reduce consumption of such
foods or replace them with healthier alternatives, as well as increasing awareness of advertising,
marketing and promotion of such foods by the media and food outlets.

6 EMOTIONAL EATING

Many people gain weight in response to stress and emotional turmoil. They use food as a way of
coping with any number of psychological issues – frustration and anger, sorrow and anxiety, even
boredom. It is a common problem, especially in people who give up smoking, but also in people who
have experienced psychologically disturbing events either as children or as adults. The answer is to
gain awareness of emotional cues to overeating while making changes to the diet that help control
appetite and limit excess calorie intake, while developing psychological strategies to overcome it.

7 INACTIVITY

This problem can occur as a result of increased reliance on cars, public transport, labour-saving
devices and home entertainment. More specifically, reduced activity may lead to weight gain
following illness or injury, changes in circumstances or job, boredom with gym attendance,
perceived cost as well as time, distance and climate constraints. The answer is to increase
activity gradually by reducing time spent in inactivity and increasing opportunistic exercise such
as walking up stairs and getting off the bus one stop earlier, before progressing to more
structured activities incorporating aerobic and strength training exercise.

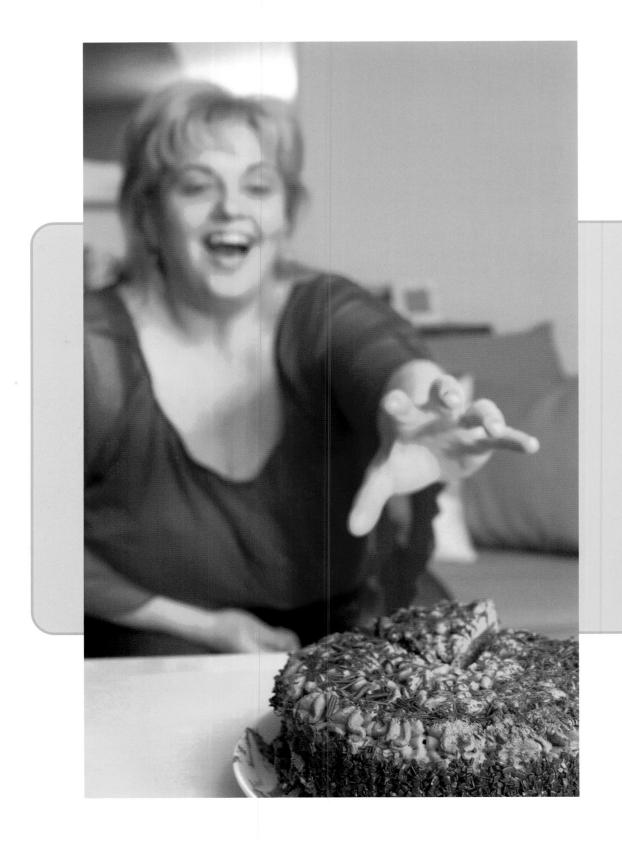

1

FOOD, ENERGY AND WEIGHT

DIETS AND DIETING

Dieting is now big business, boosted by expensive advertising and marketing campaigns promoting the latest diet plans and weight-loss products. Very often, these are aimed more at increasing sales and profits than promoting permanent weight loss,

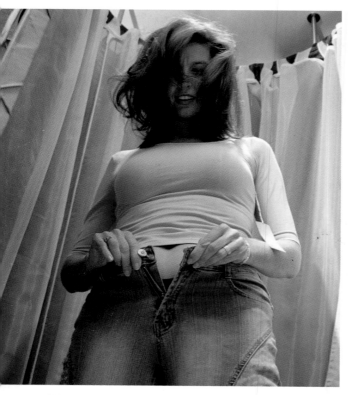

We are often made aware of the need to shed a few pounds if our clothes no longer fit. If your jeans start feeling tight about the waist, it's time to think about cutting back on the calories.

but their sales pitches are music to the ears of desperate dieters searching for a quick and easy way to lose weight.

New 'miracle' diets are constantly appearing in books, magazines and newspapers, supposedly based on some breakthrough discovery that unlocks the secret to effortless weight loss. The problem is not that none of these commercial diets is effective, but that separating the good from the bad and the downright ugly can be difficult if you lack the necessary background knowledge. You may end up simply going for the promise of painless, rapid, permanent weight loss that needs no change to your lifestyle – if you believe that such a thing is possible – especially when such promises are accompanied by anecdotal accounts and unsubstantiated 'personal testimonials', which usually claim total success.

In truth, most commercial diets will actually work if they result in a reduction in average daily calorie intake (this is true no matter what you can or cannot eat). You will lose weight if you follow these diets to the letter, but whether they are healthy or sustainable in the long term is altogether a different matter. Much of the short-term success of such diets lies in their novelty factor and/or their simplicity. You may like being told what you can and cannot eat, because it can make life so much simpler when you don't have to decide for yourself. Having a structure or 'prescription' for weight loss can also give you a feeling of empowerment and of being in control, especially if you soon start losing weight. Initial and rapid weight loss can be very motivating if you have repeatedly tried and failed in the past.

THE DIGESTIVE SYSTEM

As food travels through your system, it is broken down in various ways. The nutrients in your food are absorbed while the rest is expelled by the body as waste.

1 Mouth
The teeth break up food into manageable lumps while saliva turns them into a semi-liquid pulp and eases it down the throat.

2 Oesophagus
Food in mush-like form is pushed down this long muscular tube by the action of peristalsis, whereby muscles rhythmically contract and relax.

3 Stomach
The mechanical breakdown of food is completed here by muscular bands that churn, knead and mix the food with gastric juices.

4 Small Intestine
80 percent of nutrient absorption occurs here as does the majority of chemical digestion. Digestive juices from the liver, gallbladder and pancreas act on the food and the nutrients pass into the intestinal lining and then to the blood.

5 Large Intestine
Water and minerals are absorbed and digestive waste is expelled.

Simplifying the process of dieting is what makes restrictive diets so popular. They work by eliminating whole food groups or specific types of food, such as carbohydrates or fried foods, thereby limiting your choice of what you eat. By telling you that you cannot have these foods, the diets help you control your desire for them, and you are willing to comply (for a short time, anyway) if that means losing weight. At the same time, because you are forced to eat the same limited range of foods over and over again, you begin to lose interest in them and so you eat less of them as well, and lose more weight.

Some diets work in the opposite way, however, not by simplifying but by complicating dieting to such an extent that they require military levels of planning and execution. Inevitably, with lack of time and all the confusion, you cut out many foods for fear of eating the wrong ones and breaking your new-found diet.

This can lead to weight loss, but unfortunately any diet that is too complicated or restrictive will eventually lose its appeal, and you will abandon it out of sheer boredom. What may be distracting and fun at the beginning soon becomes monotonous and inconvenient. You start tweaking and modifying the diet to make it more acceptable, but

FAT FACT

SUCCESS WITH FORMULA DIETS

If you replace meals with nutritional shakes and bars (formula diets), they can help you to lose weight, but only when accompanied by professional nutritional and behavioural counselling. They are less successful when you attempt them on your own.

eventually you give up and discard it altogether. You crave the foods that you have had to forego, return to your old eating habits, and soon regain any weight you might have lost. Diets can also fail if they are based on poor nutritional concepts and leave you feeling hungry and lacking in energy.

YO-YO DIETING

Sometimes, even if a diet is sustainable and you manage to lose a fair amount of weight, this weight loss is not permanent. As soon as you get down to your target weight, come off the diet and go back to more manageable, 'normal' eating, you put all the weight back on again. Then you latch onto the next big diet craze and go through the whole cycle all over again.

This process of weight cycling, or yo-yo dieting, as it is often called, is not only unhealthy but can make it increasingly hard for you to reach and maintain your target weight. It may even lead to weight gain in the long run, because every cycle of weight loss and regain causes physical and mental changes that make future attempts at losing weight more difficult.

The main problem with yo-yo dieting is the way that your body reacts when you lose weight too quickly, and this reaction is a self-preservation mechanism that developed in the early stages of human evolution. If you diet too drastically, your body interprets the sharp reduction in food intake as the onset of a famine. Then, when you begin eating normally again, it starts building up its fat reserves so that it will have an energy source to draw on if the 'famine' returns.

FAT FACT

YO-YO DIETING EXPANDS YOUR WAISTLINE

On-and-off dieting may alter the distribution of fat around your body so that it becomes increasingly centred on your waist. This has implications for your health (see page 21) as well as for your appearance.

Your body cuts down its overall energy expenditure and gets better at conserving calories, and also becomes more efficient at using fat. Any fat in your food is more likely to be stored as body fat instead of being used to produce energy, and your body becomes more resistant to tapping into its own fat stores for fuel. In other words, your body learns to hang on to fat. This makes it harder for you to lose weight in the future, and you may find you that you actually gain a little weight after every dieting cycle.

Yo-yo dieting is also

DIET PATTERNS

Yo-yo dieting is characterized by fluctuating periods of weight gain and weight loss. Though steady dieting doesn't produce as much quick weight loss, it can ensure that weight loss is more permanent.

Weight

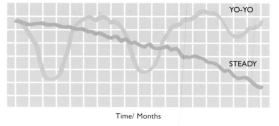

YO-YO

STEADY

Time/ Months

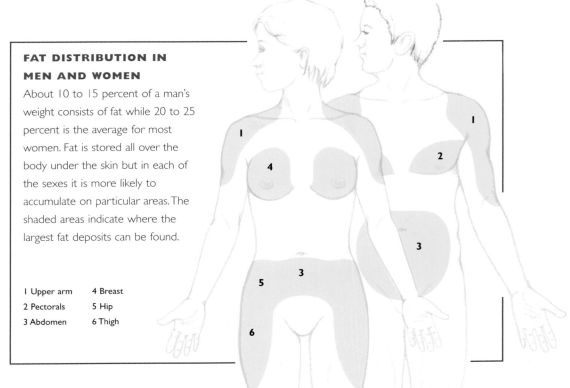

FAT DISTRIBUTION IN MEN AND WOMEN

About 10 to 15 percent of a man's weight consists of fat while 20 to 25 percent is the average for most women. Fat is stored all over the body under the skin but in each of the sexes it is more likely to accumulate on particular areas. The shaded areas indicate where the largest fat deposits can be found.

1 Upper arm   4 Breast
2 Pectorals   5 Hip
3 Abdomen   6 Thigh

counterproductive from a psychological point of view, because repeated dieting keeps your mind focused on food, especially if the diets are complicated. And a diet that restricts or forbids certain foods will only increase your cravings for them, so you are more likely to binge on them if you drop your guard or when you come off the diet. You are then in danger of falling into the trap of false starts, which happens when you start a diet but keep coming off it with the intention of restarting it after just one last binge. You then end up consuming more calories overall than if you had never started the diet at all.

Repeatedly trying and failing to achieve your ideal weight is also damaging to your motivation and morale. The constant disappointment it brings will make you feel more defeated and depressed, and you may even give up dieting altogether and actually turn to food for comfort.

Prescriptive and commercial diets, on the whole, are about quick-fix answers to long-term problems. They rarely teach nutritional skills for appetite control and lasting weight management, and in fact, many of the theories and practices they advocate are actually flawed. Some of this flawed thinking may remain in the back of your mind, even though it hasn't helped you to lose weight, and it can prevent you from moving on and making sensible changes to your diet and lifestyle in the future. Bear in mind that the best diet for you will be one that takes account of your overall lifestyle, and an optimal weight-loss diet is not the same as an optimal weight-management diet. The latter is the one that promotes better health for a longer, more fulfilling life.

As for weight-loss dietary supplements and miracle slimming aids, there is scant evidence that any of them contribute to long-term weight loss. They mostly contain either caffeine (or other appetite-suppressing stimulants) or some form of fibre that is supposed to keep you feeling full. Their side-effects are mostly unknown, and they usually come with a high price tag, making them unsuitable for long-term use.

SUCCESSFUL DIETING

If you are planning to go on a diet, bear in mind that it will only be successful if you want to lose weight for the right reasons. Without a good incentive or proper motivation, losing weight is very hard and you will find it difficult to make and maintain the lifestyle changes that will enable you to achieve your goal.

Think carefully about what you are trying to achieve by losing weight. For example, 'looking good' and 'feeling good' are goals often presented in the same sentence as if one naturally leads to the other, but you should try to separate the two in your mind. Looking good does not always lead to eternal happiness, happiness is not determined purely by how you look, and the cure for unhappiness is not necessarily weight loss.

Instead, your goal should be to improve your overall physical and mental well-being by making a healthy diet a permanent part of your lifestyle. Don't fall into the trap of playing a numbers game on the scales with quick-fix diets that inevitably lead to disappointment – a diet should not have a beginning, a middle and an end. You have to think long-term, it is the only way to step off the dieting merry-go-round.

You must also be realistic about the amount of weight you can expect to lose, and the weight you can expect to maintain. You may lose weight by cutting your calorie consumption, but you will not be able to maintain it if, for example, the calorie intake needed to do so is too low for you. As your calorie intake inevitably goes up again, so will your weight. If it is unlikely that you will ever be a size 8, perhaps you would be better off as a size 14.

SET REALISTIC TARGETS

Wanting to lose a lot of weight as fast as possible is a common ambition but it is neither realistic nor healthy. Rapid weight loss is the sure-fire way to a lifelong struggle with weight. Set long-term goals for your weight loss, but focus more on

FAT FALLACY

LOW-CARB DIETS CHANGE YOUR METABOLISM

High-protein, low-carbohydrate diets do not lead to weight loss by altering your metabolism to make it burn more fat. People on these diets lose weight simply because they eat fewer calories by cutting out most carbohydrates — including the highly refined, processed varieties — and eat a lot of animal protein, which is very filling. Such diets are rarely sustainable for very long and nor should they be, as they raise serious concerns with regard to long-term health.

short-term, achievable targets for changes to your overall lifestyle, not just to your diet.

Make small changes that you can maintain and build on, because eating in a way that you cannot foresee yourself doing in a year's time will guarantee that you remain firmly in the cycle of yo-yo dieting. Changes have to be manageable and sit comfortably with other priorities in your life because, even with the best will in the world, other demands on your life and your time may prevent you from making the necessary changes.

LEARN ABOUT NUTRITION

In an environment deluged with different weight-loss strategies, you need a good understanding of nutrition, appetite control and energy physiology if you want to find one that both suits you and really works. A good diet must help you to control your appetite and reduce your calorie intake to help you to lose weight, but must also give you enough energy and provide all your nutritional needs to ensure your long-term health (see the chart opposite).

On the whole, though, you should beware of diets based on complex scientific theories. These theories, although useful, change with progress in dietary science. As new advances are made in our understanding of appetite, nutrition, exercise and their impact on weight, that which is presented as fact today may change into fiction tomorrow.

FAT FALLACY

DETOX DIETS RAPIDLY ELIMINATE TOXINS

Detox diets do not eliminate toxins any faster than a normal healthy diet does. Your body produces toxins every day as by-products of your normal metabolism, and unless you suffer from some form of kidney, liver or bowel disorder, they are quickly eliminated. In fact, if there are any fat-soluble toxins stored in your fat cells, a sudden drop in calorie intake caused by a detox diet can actually flood your body with them. Slow weight loss with a healthy diet is a much less damaging way of eliminating toxins from your body.

ENERGY REQUIREMENTS

MEN

Age	Activity Level	Daily Calories
18-34 years	Sedentary	2510
	Active	2900
	Very Active	3350
35-64 years	Sedentary	2400
	Active	2750
	Very Active	3350
65-74 years	Sedentary	2330
75+ years	Sedentary	2100

WOMEN

Age	Activity Level	Daily Calories
18-54 years	Sedentary	1940
	Active	2150
	Very Active	2500
	Pregnant	2400
	Breastfeeding	2750
55-74 years	Sedentary	1900
	Active	2000
75+years	Sedentary	1680

WEIGHT AND HEALTH

Being overweight can harm your health, and the more overweight you are, the more your health will suffer. For example, obese adults have more hospitalizations per year, more out-patient visits, higher prescription drug costs and a lower quality of life due to ill-health. Being 20 kilograms overweight has the same risk to health as smoking 20 cigarettes per day, and the number of annual deaths due to obesity among US adults is now approximately 300,000.

During surgery, either emergency or planned, obese patients of all ages are more likely to suffer complications and to have poorer wound healing and longer recovery times. In some cases, surgery has to be postponed until the patient's weight can be sufficiently reduced. Obesity is also linked to cancer, especially cancers of the breast, large intestine, uterus, prostate, kidney, cervix and ovaries. Compared to people of normal weight, obese men are 25 percent more likely to develop cancer and obese women 37 percent more likely.

The relationship between health and body weight is complex, because either can influence the other and it can be difficult to work out which was the cause and which the effect. Often, it may be a combination of both. Just as weight gain can cause illness, some illnesses can cause weight gain directly while others cause it indirectly by stopping you from being active.

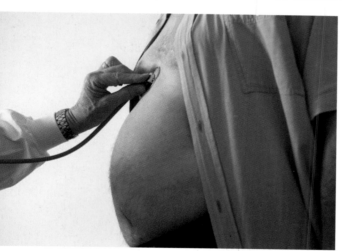

Although the latest research indicates that being overweight may not produce a shortened life span, it will, however, lead to numerous long-term health problems.

SPECIFIC HEALTH RISKS

Obesity affects almost every single organ system of the body, either directly because of the physical burden placed on it or indirectly because of the social, emotional and psychological effects of being seriously overweight.

The greatest risk to health probably comes from the added stress that obesity places on the circulation system (the heart, arteries and veins). When you are overweight, your heart has to pump harder to force blood and oxygen around your body, and it may become enlarged under pressure and then fail completely. The high pressures generated can cause narrowing of the arteries, leading to high blood pressure, which can in turn lead to kidney disease, angina, heart disease and an increased risk of heart attacks and strokes. Your veins can

CHECK YOUR BODY MASS INDEX

The usual way to assess whether a person is underweight, overweight or of normal weight is to calculate his or her body mass index (BMI), which shows the relationship between height and weight. To find your own BMI, refer to the chart below. In general, the risk of health problems increases as BMI increases above 25, and the risk of premature death increases once a BMI of 35 or over is reached. However, the BMI is not ideal because it does not differentiate between lean tissue and body fat, which is more relevant to health risks, so someone very muscular would still be classified as overweight despite having little fat. At present, though, the BMI is still the quickest way of assessing risk from excess body weight without using special equipment.

BMI READINGS
under 20 = underweight,
20-25 = healthy,
over 25 = overweight,
over 30 = clinically obese

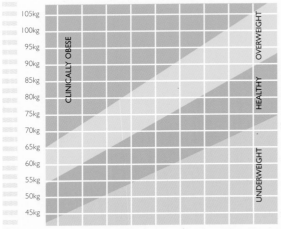

also become enlarged, which can result in unsightly varicose veins.

Becoming obese will also harm your digestive system, because when you constantly overeat, your liver and pancreas have to work harder to digest and assimilate the greater food intake. This increases the risk of liver disorders, gallstone formation and diabetes. Diabetes occurs when your pancreas starts secreting too much insulin (the hormone that regulates your blood sugar levels), and then becomes exhausted and unable to produce enough of it. In fact, obesity and diabetes go together like smoking and lung cancer and, often, insulin production problems begin up to ten years before diabetes is diagnosed.

In women, obesity can cause hormonal disturbances leading to menstrual irregularities and infertility, while in men, such disturbances can lead to lower fertility and breast enlargement. Obese people are also susceptible to a condition known as obstructive sleep apnea, which happens when a build-up of fat around the neck puts pressure on the airway during sleep. The airway becomes temporarily blocked and the person, in effect, stops breathing, resulting in a sudden awakening. This can disrupt sleep patterns and cause daytime fatigue, lack of concentration and poor memory, which are associated with increased risks of accidents. More significant, however, is the link between sleep apnea and an increased risk of heart disease. A neck circumference of more than 43 cm is thought to increase the risk of developing this condition, especially in middle-aged men.

RISKS OF BEING OVERWEIGHT

As well as the psychological problems involved in excess weight, and the greater risk of being prone to cancer, diabetes and circulatory disease, being very overweight also can have harmful physical effects on your body's organs.

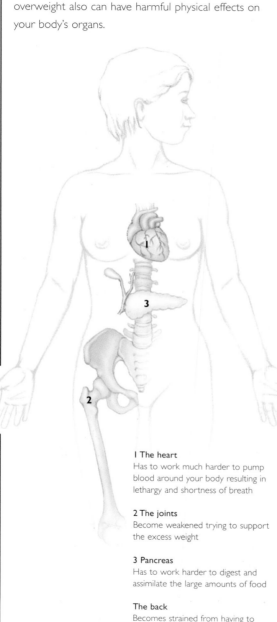

I The heart
Has to work much harder to pump blood around your body resulting in lethargy and shortness of breath

2 The joints
Become weakened trying to support the excess weight

3 Pancreas
Has to work harder to digest and assimilate the large amounts of food

The back
Becomes strained from having to support a heavy body

In both men and women, the physical pressure of excess body fat can impair the movement of the diaphragm, the sheet of muscle that expands the chest cavity to draw air into the lungs. This causes breathing difficulties that may be misdiagnosed as asthma. It also increases the risk of hiatus hernia, where the stomach is pushed up into the chest wall cavity, and of acid reflux, where acid from the stomach is forced up into the oesophagus (gullet), causing heartburn and indigestion. Excess pressure can also strain the bladder and uterus, causing stress and exercise incontinence and increase the risk of prolapse of the womb, rectum and supporting structures. Carrying excess weight also places greater pressure on the muscles and joints, leading to arthritis, joint pains, muscular strains and back pain.

THE PSYCHOLOGICAL BURDEN

Being overweight also carries with it psychological and social consequences. Obesity, unlike high blood pressure or diabetes, is a visible sign of a poor diet and inactivity, and carries the social stigmas of sloth and gluttony. As a result, many overweight individuals have to endure social prejudice. This can begin during childhood, with bullying and exclusion from many school activities, and continue into adulthood, when obesity can make it difficult to get or to keep a good job. Some industries, such as fashion and media, are particularly prone to discrimination in body size and shape. On average, obese individuals earn less than their leaner counterparts.

An obese adult may also face problems with ordinary daily activities, such as using public transport, cleaning the house and buying or trying on new clothes. Many leisure activities may be impractical, impossible or avoided out of sheer embarrassment. There is also the personal physical discomfort of being overweight. These together can have a significant effect on well-being, self-confidence and personal independence. Many of these issues can create problems within relationships, and statistics show that obese people are less likely to marry and more likely to divorce. Together, all these factors may account for the higher rates of depression and suicide recorded among the overweight population.

Unfortunately, the physical, social and psychological consequences of being overweight can create vicious cycles that exacerbate the problems because they discourage physical activity. This leads to further weight gain, and the physical discomfort and psychological impact of that may further reduce motivation for activity and increase emotional eating. The reduced opportunities for jobs, education, marriage and social inclusion may lead to lower incomes, which reduce the range of healthy choices available and the ability to take part in active sports. A low income also increases chronic stress, which can lead to comfort eating and excessive drinking.

APPLE- AND PEAR-SHAPED BODIES

As well as the levels of fat, its distribution around the body also has implications for health. Fat around the trunk or girth produces an 'apple' shape, which is commonly seen in men and is linked to a cluster of disorders including diabetes, high blood pressure, abnormal blood fats and an increased risk of heart disease. Fat distributed over the hips and thighs, the 'pear' shape, is more commonly seen in women and this appears to place women at lower risk from these disorders. After the menopause, however, women tend to accumulate fat around their abdomens and become increasingly apple-shaped. An apple shape in women is also associated with greater risk of hormone irregularities and gallstones. In general, there is an increased risk of ill-health for a man when his waist measurement rises above 95 cm, and for a woman when hers exceeds 88 cm.

SMALL LOSSES, BIG BENEFITS

Losing weight can reverse many of the harmful effects of obesity, and it doesn't have to be extensive to produce significant benefits. Reducing body weight by just 5–10 percent can produce measurable improvements in many aspects of health, including a 50 percent reduction in risk from diabetes, a 50 percent reduction in cancer risk, and a lowering of blood pressure and blood lipids (fats) and the disorders they can cause. Furthermore, improvements in mobility, self-confidence, and independence often accompany even small reductions in weight. These changes can make a huge difference to a person's quality of life – by far the best incentive to lose weight.

MEDICAL ISSUES

If you are worried about being overweight but are unable to diet successfully, it's a good idea to consult your doctor. As well as giving you useful help and advice, he or she might refer you to a specialist such as a dietitian, nutritionist or behavioural counsellor, and will probably check you for symptoms of any underlying medical condition that might be causing your problem. Such conditions include changes in hormone levels, psychological disorders, and the side effects of drugs prescribed for other disorders.

Hormones are chemicals that circulate within your body to control the functions of your glands and organs, and they can have a big effect on your moods, emotions and appetite. Unusual changes in hormone levels are associated with a number of medical conditions, including hypothyroidism (underactive thyroid gland), Cushing's disease (a disorder of the adrenal glands) and polycystic ovarian syndrome (a disorder of the ovaries). These changes can lead to weight gain by affecting your metabolism, your ability to regulate your blood sugar levels, your propensity to store fat and your body fat distribution.

Psychological disorders, especially mood disorders such as anxiety and depression (including postnatal depression), can contribute indirectly to weight gain by making you less interested in physical activity and more prone to emotional eating. Women are also at risk of weight gain if they suffer from premenstrual syndrome, which can intensify food cravings. Fluid retention, another cause of weight gain, frequently occurs in women as part of their normal

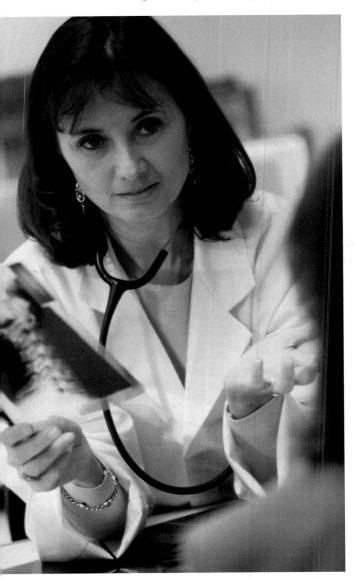

Doctors and other health-care professionals have much to offer on the subject of weight loss. They will certainly be able to tell you how your weight is affecting your general health.

menstrual cycle. It can also occur, in both men and women, as a result of circulation problems and kidney disorders.

Of the drugs that can have weight gain as a side effect, the most commonly implicated are steroids, antidepressants, blood-pressure medication, hormone replacement therapies and contraceptive pills. If you are taking any of these drugs, or any other medication (especially long term) and you are putting on weight, it may be worth discussing the problem with your doctor.

WEIGHT-LOSS DRUGS

Given the huge increase in health-threatening obesity in the West, much drug research has focused on ways of helping people to moderate their eating. As a result, there are now a number prescription drugs that can help over-eaters to regain a sense of portion size and take control of their appetites. They also boost metabolisms that may falter when calorie intake is reduced (see page 60).

Many these drugs are centrally acting appetite suppressants, which act directly on the appetite centre in the brain to reduce cravings or promote feelings of fullness. The most commonly prescribed are phentermine (Ionamin), diethylproprion (Tenuate Dospan) and sibutramine (Reductil). Phentermine and diethylproprion are for short-term use only, whereas sibutramine can be taken for up to one year.

These medicines are not intended as alternatives to adopting healthy eating habits and taking more exercise. They are an aid to achieving these goals and, ideally, should be used for only a short period of time. There are significant restrictions on the use of these drugs, which can have side effects and do not work for everyone. If you are prescribed them, you must remain under careful medical supervision throughout your treatment and work closely with your doctor to discuss the risks and benefits at every step.

Another prescription drug, orlistat (Xenical), works in a very different way. Instead of suppressing your appetite, it blocks the action of an enzyme called lipase that is involved in digesting fat in your intestines. When you eat a meal containing a significant amount of fat, orlistat will prevent about a third of the fat from being absorbed by your body. The unabsorbed fat will be removed in your bowel movements. As with appetite suppressants, there are significant restrictions on the use of orlistat and it can have unpleasant side effects, so it must only be taken under medical supervision.

FAT FALLACY

PREGNANCY MAKES YOU FAT
Although many women do gain body weight during and after pregnancy, it is usually because of lifestyle changes (more food, less exercise) and not the pregnancy itself.

GENETICS AND EARLY DEVELOPMENT

Many people who have difficulty controlling their weight often insist that being overweight simply runs in their family. They point to their parents, siblings and other relatives who are equally overweight, as evidence of their genetic inheritance. Are these people simply making excuses for their size, or can body shape and size be inherited just like other physical features or character traits? The simple answer is yes, but, as usual, it is really not as straightforward as that.

Body weight is not something you inherit directly in a physical form, like flat feet or dimples. What you do inherit is the tendency or predisposition to become overweight. Inheriting this tendency doesn't automatically guarantee that you will do so but not inheriting it doesn't mean that you can't become overweight – it all depends on other factors in your lifestyle and your environment.

Because genetic inheritance is only one of a number of factors that can act together to make you gain excess weight, becoming overweight is often described as 'multifactorial'. Among these factors, the most significant are your overall level of physical activity and the types and amounts of food that you eat.

It is thought that inheritance, as opposed to environment ('nature vs nurture'), could account for as much as 20–40 percent of final body size. This has been calculated by studying identical and nonidentical twins that have been raised together or apart, and by looking at adopted children raised apart from their biological families. By looking at variations in body size within these groups, it is possible to see to what extent their environment or genetic make-up has contributed to their weight, as some of the groups share the same environment and others share the same genetic make-up.

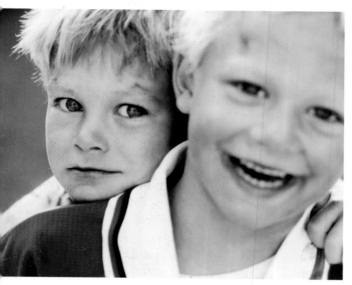

Research programmes studying identical and nonidentical twins show that inherited factors can account for 20–40 percent of the differences in body weight between otherwise similar individuals.

A number of more structured experiments also support the importance of inheritance in linking diet, exercise and body weight. When identical twins are placed on identical calorie and exercise regimes, they lose and gain similar amounts of weight. When individuals not genetically related are put on identical regimes, they show a large degree of variation in response, again by between 20–40 percent.

So what does this tell us about weight control? Most importantly, it tells us that no single specific diet or exercise regime will produce the desired result in everyone. We are all different. Just as we have different-shaped faces and bodies, we also differ in our appetites and tastes, and our capacity to burn fat, store fat, and gain muscle. So there may be some aspects of body shape that we cannot change, no matter how hard we try, and, when it comes to controlling our weight, we must appreciate that although everyone may in theory be capable of losing weight, the experience of doing so will be different for everyone, and more difficult for some people than for others.

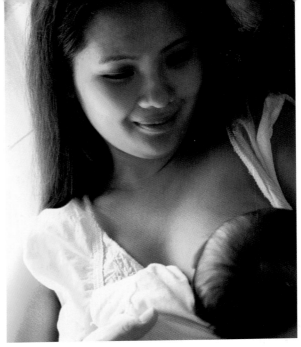

The diet of a nursing mother affects the taste of her milk, and this influences the types of food her child will prefer. A child that gets a taste for fruit and vegetables from his or her mother's milk is likely to grow up with a preference for these foods.

EARLY DEVELOPMENT

We all know that our environment can influence our weight as children and adults, but did you know that this might begin as far back as when we are embryos, growing inside the womb? The nutrition of the growing embryo can affect birth weight, and recent evidence has shown that low birth weight may lead to obesity in later life, as well as to greater risk of heart disease. At the other end of the scale, babies born with very high birth weights, often to mothers who are diabetic or obese, are equally prone to becoming obese as adults.

Early nutrition can also affect taste preferences in adulthood. The taste of the milk produced by nursing mothers depends on their diet and this can, in turn, affect the foods the infant is likely to develop a 'taste' for in later life. Nursing mothers who eat plenty of fruit and vegetables are more likely to have children who also like these foods. Those who have a diet that lacks such foods, and is high in fat and sugar, are more likely to have children that dislike the taste of fruit and vegetables and prefer fatty, sugary foods instead.

The climate into which babies are born may also influence their weight as adults. Adults born in colder climates tend to be more overweight. It may be that ambient temperatures can alter the physiology or the number of fat cells the growing embryo or infant has, making him or her more likely to lay down body fat in later life.

There is little we can do as adults to alter our genetics or early development, but perhaps it is reassuring for some people to know at least that they may have legitimate reasons for struggling more with controlling their weight than others.

METABOLIC FACTORS

We all know that our bodies need food to function, but just how does the amount you eat affect your weight? The key factor is your metabolism – all the biochemical processes taking place inside your body to keep you alive and functioning.

Your body is made up of billions of cells including bone, muscle, fat and skin cells, the cells of your internal organs, brain and nerve cells, and blood cells. Each type has a specific job but all work together. These cells' activities, occurring constantly and simultaneously around your body together, make up your metabolism. Your metabolic rate is a measure of the total metabolic activity of your body is at any given time, and it changes throughout the day. For example, it is high when you are physically active, lower when you are resting, and lower still when you are asleep.

All these metabolic activities need energy to fuel them, and this comes from energy-rich foods, such as carbohydrates (sugars and starches) and fats, that your digestive system extracts from your food. Your body converts these into simpler substances, called substrates, which your bloodstream delivers to the cells along with oxygen from the air you breathe in. These substrates include glucose, a simple type of sugar made from carbohydrates, and forms of fat made from the fats in your food.

Within the cells, chemical reactions combine the substrates with the oxygen, releasing the energy the cells need and producing heat, carbon dioxide and water. The heat helps to maintain your body's internal temperature, while your bloodstream carries the carbon dioxide and water away to your lungs, where they are expelled from your body in the air you breathe out. Your metabolism is therefore said to 'burn' the energy in food because, like a fire, it too requires oxygen and releases heat.

The sources of energy in food vary according to whether the food is of plant or animal origin, but there are four main types: fat, protein, carbohydrate and alcohol. All of these can be broken down by the digestive system to produce substrates, although the body has many other uses for them apart from energy production. The energy they contain is measured in kilojoules or, more commonly, in calories, and the total number of calories in a given amount of food will depend on how much of these substances it contains.

Fat, the most energy-dense constituent of food, provides 9 calories of energy per gram. Protein and carbohydrate each provide 4 calories per gram, while a gram of alcohol provides 7 calories. Food also provides a number of vitamins, minerals and other substances essential for optimal cell functioning and metabolism, and so has nutritional value as well as just calories or calorific value.

STORING ENERGY

When the food you eat contains more energy than you need, your body stores the surplus for later use. It does this in two main ways. The first is by converting some of the excess glucose into a substance called glycogen, and storing it in the liver and muscles where it can be quickly converted back into glucose again when needed (see pages 56–7). The second is by converting most of the surplus fat, plus the rest of the excess glucose, into body fat, and storing this inside your fat cells as a long-term energy reserve. One kilo of body fat stores approximately 3500 calories of energy.

This system of energy storage is essential, because metabolism occurs continuously (even when you are asleep) but food intake does not. However, if you regularly eat more food than your body needs, you will keep storing the extra calories as fat and gain weight. If you regularly eat less than your body needs, though, you will lose weight.

YOU AND YOUR METABOLISM

If you want to lose weight, you either have to increase your metabolic rate or reduce your energy input (see box, right). Ideally, you should do both. This principle forms the basis of all effective weight-loss diets.

So what controls your metabolic rate and your tendency to gain weight? The most important factor is your genetic make-up (see pages 24–5). Your genes influence your body size and shape, and the amount and distribution of fat and lean muscle tissue. Generally, the larger or taller you are, the more cells there are in your body and so the greater will be your metabolic rate. This is especially the case if you have more lean muscle tissue than fat tissue, because muscle is much more metabolically active than fat.

THE ENERGY BALANCE EQUATION

Our weight is a reflection of the balance between the energy (calories) we consume and the energy we use. Our energy intake is determined by the amount and type of food we eat. Our energy expenditure is determined by a combination of our resting metabolic rate (RMR) and the amount of calories we burn in day-to-day activities.

The resting metabolic rate is the amount of energy needed just to keep your body ticking over, like the fuel used by a car when the engine is idling. Even if you stayed in bed all day, you'd still need to use large amounts of energy just to maintain your body's normal functions. In most people, RMR accounts for between half and three-quarters of the energy required each day. The other component is the amount of energy you expend in exercise and everyday activity.

If energy intake equals energy expenditure, body weight will remain stable, but if intake exceeds expenditure, the excess energy is stored as fat.

Eating just a small amount in excess of your needs will result in a slow but steady weight gain. To lose weight, you simply need to tip the balance so that you use more calories than you consume; in this situation the body will draw on fat reserves to provide the energy it needs. You can do this by restricting the number of calories you eat or by increasing the amount of calories you use, but without a doubt the best way is by a combination of both – diet and exercise.

In fact, muscle burns up nearly ten times more calories per kilo than fat does, so just having more lean tissue, at whatever weight you are, means you will burn more calories even when you are resting. So as far as your metabolic rate is concerned, your body composition is as important, if not more important, than your body weight.

Your body's ability to burn fat for fuel is yet another factor that is, to a certain extent, under genetic control. Some people are genetically better than others at conserving fat. Whether the fat comes from their diet or from their body's own fat stores, they are more 'fat-sparing' and fuel-efficient, and so they gain weight more easily and lose weight with greater difficulty.

Two more factors that heavily influence your metabolic rate are your gender and your age. Women on the whole, have lower metabolic rates than men because of differences in size and muscle tissue, and in hormones, some of which can affect the rate at which the body burns energy. Your metabolism also slows down with advancing age, regardless of your gender, so as you get older you have to eat less food just to stay at the same weight, and it becomes harder to lose weight.

Your metabolic rate will also rise or fall in response to certain situations. For example, it will rise whenever your body is placed under any kind of stress. This includes not only emotional and psychological stress but also the stress of physical activity. Exertion, or simply movement of any kind (even standing instead of sitting) requires muscle contractions, which use up energy. The greater the physical activity, the greater will be your energy expenditure and thus the rise in your metabolic rate. Even fidgeting burns calories! Physical activity also increases the amount of lean muscle tissue your body contains and this can help boost your resting metabolic rate, the rate at which your body uses up energy while you are resting.

Anything that leads to loss or wasting of muscle tissue, however, will reduce your metabolic rate. This can result from prolonged inactivity, perhaps due to illness or injury, but another important cause is prolonged fasting that leads to sudden and rapid weight loss. Your body normally loses some muscle as well as fat when you lose weight, but a sudden reduction in calorie intake makes your body try to reserve as many calories as possible for your essential organs, such as your brain. It then begins to shed

RAISING YOUR METABOLIC RATE

Regular exercise strengthens the heart, lungs and muscles so that food is converted more efficiently into energy. This raises your metabolic rate. To keep your weight down, you must ensure that your daily calorie intake does not exceed your energy output. But through exercise, you can increase your calorie intake.

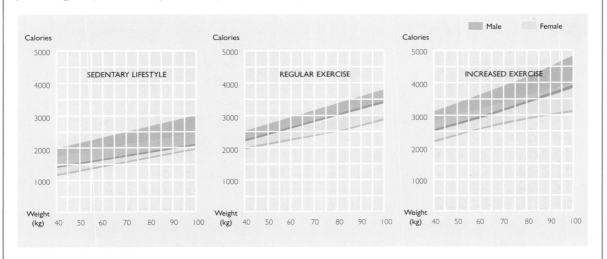

tissue that is not vital for survival but is metabolically expensive because it uses up a lot of calories. Because muscle burns about ten times more calories than fat tissue it costs your body more, in terms of energy, to hang onto muscle rather than fat, and so during rapid weight loss you lose a greater proportion of muscle tissue. Going for long periods without eating also changes your hormone levels, which further lowers your metabolic rate as well as making your body more fat-sparing and energy-efficient. Periods of prolonged fasting followed by feasting will change the composition of your body because it increasingly loses muscle while hanging onto fat.

This pattern of eating can make your body so sensitive to any drops in calorie intake that it will respond to them by lowering your metabolic rate more quickly. This can make it easier to gain weight in the future and harder to lose it because each cycle of weight loss followed by regain places your body at a greater metabolic disadvantage. So if you want to lose weight permanently you must do it slowly, avoid the temptation to enter prolonged periods of fasting, and do plenty of muscle-preserving exercise.

FAT FALLACY

OBESE PEOPLE REGULARLY EAT LARGE AMOUNTS OF FOOD

Although this is true in some cases, most people actually gain weight from small excesses in their daily food intake over a long period of time. An extra 60 calories (one small biscuit) per day is all you need to gain one kilo of fat (3500 calories) in a couple of months, and potentially over 6 kg in just one year.

PASSIVE OVERCONSUMPTION

Some people gain weight because they regularly overeat without being aware of it, and without any active intent or desire to do so. This process, called passive overconsumption, is a major cause of obesity in developed countries.

WHAT CAUSES IT?

The passive overconsumer neither intends nor particularly wants to overeat, and does so without knowing it. You can easily become one if you are unaware of (or ignore) the calorie content of the foods you eat, and end up making poor dietary choices that eventually lead to weight gain.

You risk being a passive overconsumer when much of what you eat is convenience foods and you pay no attention to their calorie content, or when information about the calories in your food is unavailable, as is the case when you eat in restaurants. Handing control over what you eat to third parties such as food manufacturers, retailers and restaurateurs, and relying solely on them to determine the quality and quantity of your meals, is when your weight management problems are likely to begin.

Many people eat out or rely on prepared food bought in supermarkets to some extent, and it is easy to see why. Busy lifestyles and long working hours mean that few are able or willing to prepare their own meals, and the choice and ready availability of tasty, affordable meals seems to offer a better use of their time, money and energy. Using ready-made meals and eating out, for pleasure, convenience or out of necessity, has become the norm for many of us.

Even if you are well-informed and well-intentioned, manufacturers and retailers can still frustrate your attempts at being a more proactive consumer by giving misleading, difficult-to-interpret or downright false information about their foods. Most restaurants also offer little or no nutritional information about the food they serve, something you will be aware of if you've ever tried asking the waiter how a particular dish is made.

THE CONSEQUENCES

Many convenience foods are produced with little or no concern for their calorific or nutritional value. They are made to appeal to our eyes and our palates, and so are high in hidden fats and refined carbohydrates and low in natural fibre, making them very calorie-dense. These foods can severely restrict your ability to control calorie intake because they bypass your body's natural mechanisms for regulating food intake.

For example, foods that lack fibre are easy to chew, so you can take in a lot of calories very quickly. Because they lack bulk, you can comfortably eat large amounts of them before you feel full, by which time you will have consumed a large number of calories. The feeling of

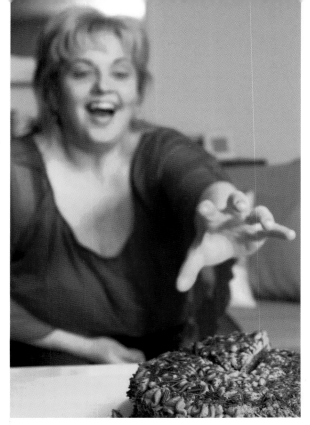

Convenience foods are designed to appeal to all our senses of sight and smell as well as taste. Specialists in the field ensure that such products are, in a sense, 'eye candy'.

NUTRITIONAL VALUES OF SOME FAST FOODS

Many fast food meals are very high in fat but low in other nutrients. Some contain no nutrients at all. Although fatty fast foods supply a lot of energy, by eating them you will be using up your calorie 'allowance' but not getting the nutrients you need to maintain good health. This is even more true of the 'empty' calories of cola.

Food	Calories	Fat(g)	Cholesterol (mg)
Bacon and egg sandwich	427	22.7 g	246 mg
2 pieces extra crispy chicken	544	37 g	168 mg
Cola, 350 ml (12 fl oz)	136	12.2 g	0 mg
Quarter-pound burger	193	0 g	61 mg
Cheese-and-tomato pizza slice	235	11.8 g	16 mg
Milk shake, 350 ml (12 fl oz)	444	14 g	42 mg
Chips, regular size	280	15.5 g	0 mg
Croissant	200	11 g	30 mg
Macaroni cheese 280 g (10 oz)	420	20 g	30 mg
Sausage roll	280	18 g	27 mg
Cheese nachos 200 g (7 oz)	814	46 g	0 mg

fullness, one of your body's natural defences against weight gain, is not triggered quickly enough and is totally overwhelmed by the number of calories reaching the intestine in such a short time. In addition, such energy-dense foods are often very tasty so they stimulate your appetite, maintaining your desire to keep right on eating even well after you are full.

Consuming such foods on a regular basis can therefore increase your overall daily calorie intake without setting off any of your internal alarm systems. This makes it easy for you to gain weight without ever realizing that you are overeating.

EATING WITHOUT THINKING

Because Michael (see page 30) relied on third parties to provide his meals, he had given them control of the quantity as well as the quality of the food he was eating. We tend to eat the portions we are given, so when he was presented with a plate of food he tended to eat it all, especially if it was delicious and not very filling. When he ate a ready-made meal or dined in a restaurant, it was the manufacturer or restaurateur who decided the portion size, and he ate what they gave him. However, one size does not fit all, and if it was more than he needed, he overate without being aware that he was doing so.

Excessive drinking, whether for reasons to do with work or when socializing with friends, had added to Michael's problem of passive overconsumption. Like many people, he was quite unaware that alcoholic drinks can add large numbers of calories to an individual's daily intake. Many bars and pubs now serve beers and wines that have a high alcohol content, and exotic cocktails that are laden with sugar and occasionally fat, making them very high in calories. It is now quite possible for a couple of drinks to give you the calorie equivalent of a burger and fries.

Looking through Michael's food diary, it quickly became apparent what his problem was, and once it was explained to him he realized that he would have to get a grip on his eating and drinking habits if was to shed the weight he had gained. What he needed was a recovery programme that would help him to choose his food more carefully, and steer him away from his reliance on restaurants and ready-made meals.

FAT FACT

HOW BEER CAN BLOAT YOUR BELLY

Beers, lagers and other fizzy drinks can overstretch the walls of your stomach and intestines, so that eventually they become less sensitive and require more and more food before they trigger the feeling of fullness. This is what, over time, will give you a beer belly. Such drinks should be avoided if possible. A glass or two of red wine is a better alternative because it's non-fizzy and contains a high concentration of health-promoting substances, such as antioxidants that help to protect your body cells from damage.

Passive Overconsumption Recovery Programme

I BECOME A PROACTIVE CONSUMER

Taking proactive measures to get more control over what you are eating isn't always easy, but it's the only way to regulate your food intake if most of your meals are made by third parties. The first step is to gain a firm understanding of the basic principles of food, nutrition and energy balance in the body, and to get to know the energy values of common foods. As tedious as this may sound, if you don't know what different foods contain and how they can affect your weight, any changes you make to your diet will be likely to fail because they are based more on guesswork than sound judgement.

You also need to familiarize yourself with the ingredients of your favourite convenience foods and learn how to read and interpret food labels. These are vital skills to develop if you are to make better food choices when shopping in supermarkets (see pages 150–55). By checking the ingredient lists and other information on food labels, you can track down those hidden fats and sugars that account for your excess calorie intake. The numbers will

FAT FALLACY

LOW-FAT FOODS ARE LESS FATTENING

Which food is less fattening: fat-free frozen yogurt or standard vanilla ice cream? The answer may surprise you because the ice cream actually turns out to be lower in calories. The reason is that much of the fat in so-called low-fat, fat-free or 'lite' foods is replaced by sugar, making the overall calorie content only marginally less or much the same as the original.

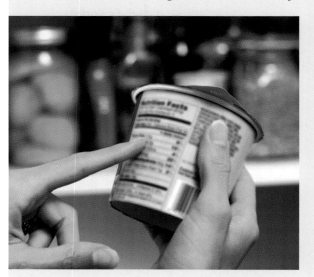

probably surprise you. Cut out these 'empty' calories – calories from ingredients that provide energy but little else of nutritional value – and you will be able to lose weight without feeling hungry or deprived.

Being proactive also means paying greater attention to your choice of food when you eat out or buy takeaway meals. Of course, there are occasions when eating out should be seen as a treat and so concerns about the nutritional value of the food can be put aside. But if you have to eat out regularly (perhaps as part of your job), then knowing whether a particular meal is high in, for example, fat or sugar, is important. Many fast-food chains now provide such nutritional information in an attempt to counteract criticisms levelled at them about this very problem, but the majority of restaurants, cafes and takeaways still do not.

Choosing wisely in a restaurant can make a substantial difference to your daily energy intake, and to make the best choices when eating out you need to acquire skills in 'menu translation'. This involves looking for key culinary terms that suggest the likely ingredients and give clues to the energy content of particular meals. For example, any food described on a menu as being deep-fried is likely to contain more fat than a similar dish that is steamed (see page 135).

Portion control is another important skill to develop if you want to continue using convenience foods and eating out. As we have seen, many of these foods can bypass your body's natural ability to control the amount of food you eat, so you will need to pay greater attention to portion sizes and apply more mindful restraint over how much you eat.

Becoming more proactive as a consumer takes time and effort, and can occasionally make you appear and feel like a member of the 'food police'. You may feel uncomfortable hanging around the aisles of a supermarket studying the food labels, or embarrassed to ask awkward questions in a restaurant, but you must overcome these barriers if you are to make the necessary changes to your diet.

GUIDELINES FOR SAFE DRINKING

Official guidelines recommend that women drink no more than three units of alcohol a day and men no more than four – one unit is half a pint of beer, or a glass of wine, or a single shot of spirits. In addition, men should drink no more than 21 units a week and women no more than 14, and both should not drink at all on at least two days per week. It is best to avoid alcohol in pregnancy.

2 BACK TO BASICS

If there is one skill that is going to help you to lose weight and keep off the pounds for life, it is the ability to prepare and cook your own meals and snacks. Cooking simple but tasty dishes from basic ingredients is the best way of knowing and controlling your food intake and reducing your reliance on convenience foods and restaurant meals. As a bonus, freshly made foods retain more of their nutrients and you will avoid any of the additives and chemicals that go into pre-prepared foods.

By choosing the right foods and preparing and cooking them appropriately (see page 135), you can regain control over your appetite, cravings, energy levels and weight. Furthermore, as your cooking improves, you may find that it is saving you money and even providing a source of stress relief. Cooking healthy food is not only good for your body and brain, but also can in time be transformed into a channel for recreation and creativity.

3 LIMIT YOUR DRINKING

Reduce your alcohol intake, if it is excessive, because this is will not only reduce your calorie intake but also help to control your appetite – alcohol makes you hungry. Stick to the recommended guidelines for sensible drinking and avoid high-calorie sugary cocktails.

PRACTICAL TIPS

Eat more slowly. It takes approximately twenty minutes for satiety (fullness) signals to reach the appetite centre in your brain and register the feeling of fullness. By slowing down your eating, you are more likely to feel full before you have taken in too many calories.

• A number of websites now list the nutritional content of the foods served at many popular fast-food outlets, including the fat, sugar and calorie content, so use this information to help you when deciding where and what to eat when out.

• Order a salad as a starter in restaurants. A salad is not only low in calories (as long as there is no high-calorie dressing) but will also make you feel fuller sooner when you are eating your main course.

• Drink a glass or two of water while waiting for your meal in a restaurant. Again, this will help you to feel fuller sooner.

• When drinking out, alternate your alcoholic drinks with either fruit juice or water to reduce your alcohol intake.

• Add your own fresh vegetables to convenience meals. This will provide more nutrients and bulk out the ready-made food, helping you to eat less of it.

PORTION CONTROL

It doesn't take all that much to cut down on the calories by eliminating or reducing food on the plate. By removing the ice cream from the pie and cutting back on the wine and the meat, the dinner has lost 500 calories.

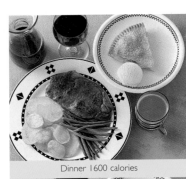

Dinner 1600 calories

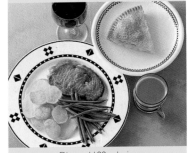

Dinner 1100 calories

EXERCISE

An adequate level of physical exercise is an essential part of a healthy lifestyle. Regular exercise, even something as simple as a brisk half-hour walk every day, improves your circulation and your immune system, helps to keep you mentally alert, and burns up calories that might otherwise end up as unwanted body fat. If you are trying to lose weight, exercise will play a key role by boosting your metabolic rate and maintaining or increasing the amount of lean muscle tissue in your body. In addition, a number of studies have found that exercise can improve your appetite regulation, which is useful both during weight loss and for long-term weight management (see pages 122–7).

Any physical exercise involves using your muscles to move or work against a load, and in your normal daily activities this load is mainly your body weight, which your muscles and bones support and carry. Your muscles are made up of specialized cells that contract (shorten) to maintain your posture, stabilize your joints and produce movement. These muscle contractions are powered by energy from the food you eat and oxygen from the air that you breathe in (see page 37).

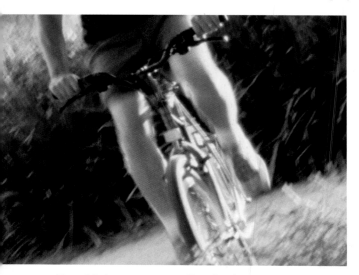

No weight-loss programme will work unless your exercise level is increased. As well as helping you to lose weight, exercise can improve body shape and lift your mood.

So how can exercise help you lose weight? When you take more exercise, your muscles have to contract harder and more often and so they use more energy, but when the levels of glucose and fats circulating in your blood are not enough to provide this energy, your body turns to its fat stores for fuel. If the amount of energy you use every day is greater than the amount you take in (in your food), then your body will have to draw on its fat stores and over time this will reduce your body fat.

Physical activity also makes your muscles stronger and bigger, so it increases the overall amount of lean tissue in your body at the same time as reducing the amount of body fat. Lean tissue burns more calories per kilo than body fat does, so with more muscle and less fat your body will use up more calories, even while you are resting. When you diet to lose weight, your metabolic rate – the rate at which you use energy – may drop because your body loses lean tissue as well as fat, but exercising can reverse this process and so prevent your metabolic rate from dropping too far.

AEROBIC AND ANAEROBIC EXERCISE

During moderate exercise, your muscles use more oxygen as well as more energy. To meet this demand for more oxygen, your body releases adrenaline and other hormones into your bloodstream to stimulate your heart and lungs to work harder, and to open up the arteries that carry oxygen-rich blood to your heart and muscles. This form of exercise, which includes brisk walking, cycling and swimming, is referred to as aerobic or cardiovascular exercise.

'Aerobic' exercise means that your muscles use up oxygen when you perform it, and 'cardiovascular' means that your heart and circulatory system play a key part in it. Regular aerobic exercise can strengthen your heart and lungs and improve blood flow, which lowers your blood pressure and reduces your risk of heart disease.

When your body cannot supply oxygen fast enough, as happens during high-intensity cardiovascular exercise such as fast running, then a degree of anaerobic (oxygen-free) metabolic activity occurs within your muscles. During anaerobic exercise, your muscles have to use a lot of extra energy in a very short time, but they can't get enough oxygen for this, they can't use up all the glucose in your bloodstream because your brain needs it, and there isn't time to draw on your stores of body fat. So they have to get the extra energy by burning up glycogen (the form in which glucose is stored in the muscles and liver), and they convert it into energy without using oxygen. The biochemical reactions involved in this create lactic acid as a by-product, and the lactic acid causes muscular pain and the runners' 'stitch'. Fatigue usually sets in quickly as the glycogen runs out and the lactic acid builds up, but when you slow down and there is enough oxygen in your bloodstream to meet your muscles' needs, your body will neutralize the lactic acid and remove it from them.

This form of intense cardiovascular exercise usually stimulates your appetite, because your body's stores of glycogen are small and quickly run out. When they do so, your body replenishes them with glucose from your bloodstream, so your blood sugar levels fall and this triggers hunger.

With less intense activity, however, your muscles use some glycogen but your body has more time to make fat available from its fat stores. This type of exercise does not use up too much

HOW EXERCISE IMPROVES YOUR MOOD

During exercise, your body produces adrenaline and feel-good brain chemicals called endorphins, and boosts levels of the neurotransmitter serotonin in your brain. The combined effects of these help to reduce stress, improve your mood, enhance your self-esteem and keep you motivated. Exercise also increases your sense of achievement and of being in control, empowering you to make and stick to changes in your lifestyle, and by keeping your mind on the present it can help you avoid negative thought patterns that can lead to anxiety and depression.

FITNESS COMPONENTS OF DIFFERENT ACTIVITIES

Sport	Muscular Strength	Aerobic Stamina	Muscular Stamina	Flexibility
Aerobic class		✔	✔	✔
Dancing	✔	✔	✔	✔
Circuit training	✔	✔	✔	✔
Walking		✔	✔	
Running		✔	✔	
Rowing	✔	✔	✔	✔
Swimming	✔	✔	✔	✔
Martial arts	✔		✔	✔
Downhill skiing		✔		
Gymnastics	✔		✔	✔
Racquets sports		✔	✔	✔
Golf		✔		
Cycling		✔	✔	

oxygen so your muscle metabolism remains aerobic, and muscle fatigue does not develop as quickly so you can keep going for longer. Your glycogen stores are not used up, so the exercise will not stimulate your appetite, and your body continues to burn some fat over the subsequent 24 hours in order to refill its glycogen stores.

Moderate aerobic exercise is particularly good for reducing abdominal fat and is the best type of exercise for promoting weight loss. Extended post-exercise fat burning also occurs with intense cardiovascular exercise, but overall its benefits are hampered by the more immediate effect on your appetite and food intake.

RESISTANCE TRAINING

One form of anaerobic exercise, however, can help you when you are trying to lose weight. Called resistance training, it targets specific muscle groups and makes them work against a load, using slow, controlled movements. It usually involves lifting weights or using your body weight against gravity, and taken to

STAYING FIT AND STAYING SLIM

Studies have found that as people improve their endurance and are able to continue exercising for longer, they increase their capacity to use fat as a source of fuel, both during exercise and at rest. However, this effect is not permanent: once you stop, the beneficial effects of exercise on your metabolism are lost. So for weight management and better health, increased physical activity must be a long-term commitment and life change – if you let up, you go up!

the extreme it is the sport of body-builders. It is anaerobic because it relies on muscle glycogen as fuel, but because it involves only short bursts of very intense activity, it doesn't empty your glycogen stores so it won't stimulate your appetite.

Resistance training is particularly effective at increasing muscle mass so it can prevent the loss of lean tissue that occurs during weight loss. It is particularly helpful for women, because they tend to have less muscle tissue than men to begin with and it diminishes with age, making weight loss more and more difficult. If you have yo-yo dieted in the past, you may have lost a substantial amount of lean tissue in the process. Resistance training can help restore some of that loss and improve the appearance of your body.

Exercise generally, but resistance training in particular, is especially valuable as you age, preventing the vicious cycle of reduced mobility and loss of muscle tissue that can occur. The thinning of bones (osteoporosis) that afflicts women after the menopause can also be reduced with resistance training, and it will help to stabilize joints and reduce arthritic pain by strengthening the surrounding muscles. It can also restore your posture and increase your core body strength, balance and physical stamina, making it a useful addition to cardiovascular exercise for promoting fat loss, improving your mobility and enhancing your quality of life.

ENERGY OUTPUT

SPORT/ACTIVITY	KJ (CAL) PER MINUTE
READING	5.5 (1.3)
WASHING UP	8.4 (2)
RAKING	8.4–10.5 (2–2.5)
OFFICE WORK	10.5 (2.5)
WALKING	4.2–14.7 (1–3.5)
SWEEPING	4.2–16.8 (1–4)
SCRUBBING	4.2–16.8 (1–4)
VACUUM CLEANING	4.2–21 (1–5)
HIKING	16.8–21 (4–5)
DIGGING	16.8–23.1 (4–5.5)
WEEDING	16.8–23.1 (4–5.5)
GOLF	16.8–25.2 (4–6)
TENNIS	25.2–33.6 (6–8)
CYCLING	42–50.4 (10–12)
SWIMMING	21–63 (5–15)
RUNNING	33.6–63 (8–15)

All activities listed are examples of kilojoule or calorie burners, helping you to keep fit and shed excess weight.

STRETCHING EXERCISES

It's important to balance muscle contraction with stretching and lengthening exercises. Without this, your muscles can shorten and stiffen, and eventually they will lose their flexibility and prevent your joints from going through their full range of motion. Stretching also can improve your posture, coordination and balance.

Stretching after exercise increases the blood flow to your muscles, which helps your body to clear them of accumulated waste products and toxins. This can reduce muscular pain and tension and the likelihood of sustaining sports-related injuries. Stretching also helps to relax muscles made tight and tense by day-to-day stress.

GRAZING

'Grazing' is a term used to describe the behaviour of someone who eats small amounts of food throughout the day instead of (or sometimes as well as) eating regular meals at specific times.

WHAT CAUSES IT?

Grazing, or constant snacking, used to be seen mainly in people who spend a lot of their time around food, such as those in the catering trade, but now it's becoming more common among the population as a whole. This is partly a reflection of our changing lifestyles and attitudes to eating. With so many responsibilities and commitments, personal and professional, more and more people are snacking on-the-go rather than taking the time to have proper sit-down meals. As the demands on our time have increased, eating while running errands, working on the computer, or in and around meetings, would seem to be a more efficient use of our time.

Our food-to-go culture has also been fuelled by the sheer amount and variety of manufactured snack foods that are now available. They are convenient, tasty and need little or no preparation other than unwrapping, and you can eat them while getting on with other things. Once, the available snacks were mainly sweets and crisps, but you can now get almost anything to eat while on the move, from breakfast replacement bars and pastries to sticks of cheese and cartons of soup. Given the investment that snack-food manufacturers make in marketing, promoting and advertising these products to us, it is little wonder that we find them so irresistible.

THE CONSEQUENCES

There are several reasons why this type of continuous eating, as opposed to having regular proper meals, can lead to weight gain. From a purely physiological view, eating small amounts of food more frequently may mean that you never feel hungry, but equally you never really feel full. The feeling of satiety (physical fullness) and satisfaction is an important signal that switches off your appetite centre, the area of your brain that controls your desire to eat. If you don't feel full after eating, your appetite centre remains switched on so you will just want to keep on eating. A short time after one snack, you will want another and then another and then another. In these circumstances, it becomes very difficult to control your appetite and it is also very easy to lose track of the quantity of food you are eating.

Eating on-the-go can also leave you feeling unsatisfied on a psychological level. When you eat while doing other things, you can't pay attention to your food and enjoy it properly, so you are more likely to underestimate the amount of food you've actually had.

Another reason that eating in this way causes weight gain has to do with the quality of the snack foods themselves. People tend to snack on manufactured foods that are highly processed and lacking in natural fibre, but laden with highly palatable fats and refined sugars. Palatability keeps your appetite switched on, but these foods are not filling so there is no fullness signal to switch it off again, so you tend to keep on snacking. High-fat, sugary snacks also stimulate your body to produce more insulin. This can lead to unstable blood sugar levels that make your cravings for such snacks even greater (see pages 52–4), and excessive insulin production can lead to more body-fat storage. These problems are less likely if you snack on low-calorie, high-fibre foods such as fruit and vegetables.

GAINING AWARENESS OF INTAKE

Margaret (see page 40) was constantly snacking while looking after her children and attending to her studies, but she never felt that she was overeating because the snacks she ate were not filling. If anything, she thought she was under-eating, as she sometimes felt quite drained of energy and put that down to a lack of food. She had struggled to lose weight because she didn't feel she could eat any less, and until she

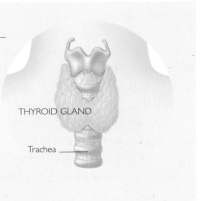

THE THYROID GLAND AND WEIGHT

An underactive or overactive thyroid gland can occasionally — in about 1 percent of the population — lead to some weight problems. The thyroid gland, which is situated at the front of the neck, produces hormones that help to regulate the body's energy levels. The correct production of thyroid hormones is crucial for promoting normal physical growth and for controlling metabolic rate.

THYROID GLAND

Trachea

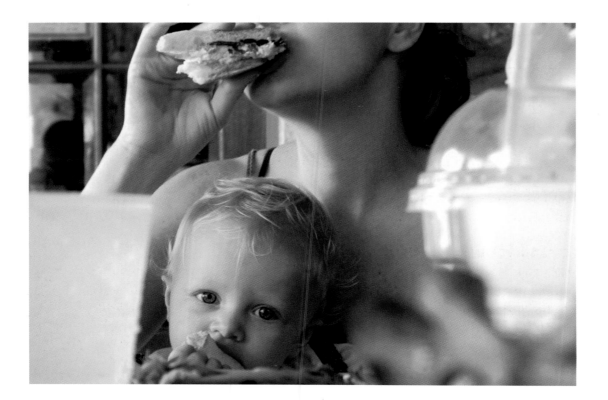

It can be very hard to take note of what and how much you eat on a daily basis – particularly if you have other things on your mind or a busy lifestyle.

began noting down everything she ate, she didn't realize quite how many calories she was consuming in a day. Even though she was quite active and had only one main meal a day (her dinner), her total daily calorie intake was surprisingly high and clearly much more than she needed.

Margaret's problem is not uncommon, but there are some people who have other, more subtle, psychological reasons for eating little and often. For example, they may feel guilty if they eat, say, a bar of chocolate all in one go. They prefer to eat it piece by piece over the course of the day so that, in a sense, they can discount it. But the chocolate bar still has the same calories, whether eaten bit by bit throughout the day or all in one go. The idea is that 'one small piece won't hurt', but it certainly can when lots of those small pieces add up to a whole bar by the end of the day.

Grazing Recovery Programme

1 FIND THE CAUSE

If you have slipped into the habit of grazing and want to get out of it, the first step you have to take is to ask yourself why it is that you are eating in this way. Is it for purely practical reasons to do with your time and commitments, or are there psychological reasons for it? Practical reasons will have purely practical solutions, but psychological reasons – such as kidding yourself that small but often is not fattening – will call for a rethink of your attitude towards food.

2 SET REGULAR MEAL TIMES

To overcome a grazing habit, your main aim should be to set regular times for meals, and to restrict your eating to those meal times. When a meal is finished, your eating should be over until the next planned meal time. This may mean eating three larger meals a day, with small snack-sized 'meals' in between them, or five smaller meals over the course of a day, but your eating must be restricted to these set times as much as possible.

At the outset, establishing these regular and specific eating times is much more important than trying to restrict your calorie intake – that's something you can tackle when you've regularized your eating times. Eating at planned intervals will help you to become more aware of the quantity of food you are eating, and help you to learn to associate hunger cues with these times.

If you are finding it difficult to stick to set meal times, then begin by having set times for snacks so that these, at least, fall into a regular pattern. When you get used to the idea of eating at specific times only, you can go on to replace your snacks with more structured meals.

You must also become more aware of, and listen to, your own body's natural hunger and satiety signals. Get into the habit of asking yourself whether you really do feel hungry every time you are about to eat, because this will help you to limit your eating to your planned meal times. Similarly, finish eating when you are comfortably full (see pages 50–51), as this will make it easier for you to control your portion sizes.

3 TIME MANAGEMENT

If you are going to succeed in changing your eating behaviour, you must make regular meal times a priority and make space for them in your daily activities. Many people think they have so many other things to do that they simply can't set aside the time for a proper meal, but often it is a lack of forward planning that is to blame (see page 126). It can also be counterproductive.

For example, taking scheduled lunch breaks at work will not only improve your mental focus and concentration, but also give you more energy so that you can return

THE PERILS OF PALATABILITY

The palatability of food, especially when it is sweet-tasting, has been shown to stimulate insulin secretion in the body regardless of the actual sugar or fat content of the food, and before the food has even reached the intestines. In other words, your body prepares itself for the calories it thinks it is about to receive by secreting insulin beforehand – and insulin not only controls your blood sugar levels, it also activates your fat-storage mechanism. So even if you try to cut your calorie intake by using artificial sweeteners and fat substitutes, your body may still react by going into fat-storage mode if the food tastes delicious. It is therefore better to avoid sweet, manufactured snacks, even if they are made with artificial sweeteners and are lower in calories, and go for natural, unadulterated whole fruits and snacks.

to work with all cylinders firing. You will also find you can work better beforehand, knowing you are going to have a break soon. Whether working at the office, in front of a computer at home or supervising your children's playtime, you will achieve much more in the day if you set time aside for relaxation and a sit-down meal. It means working smarter, not harder.

Another important part of time management involves planning what you are going to eat in advance. If you do so, you won't end up rushing around at the last minute, trying hurriedly to decide what you want to eat or even what you can eat, when you are already feeling hungry. It is at those times when you are likely to give up and go for the easier – and less healthy and probably more fattening – option of grabbing a snack. If cooking is not an option, then keep your food choices simple but always have them ready, for instance by making up a packed lunch to take to work the following day. Alternatively shop ahead for the things you will need, such as salad ingredients and cold meats, which can be bought ready-prepared so that all you need to do at the last minute is put them together to make a meal.

4 ENJOY YOUR MEAL

When you eat a meal, sit down, away from distractions, and take your time over it. Don't rush your food, or try to do anything else while you are eating (not even watching TV). Give your full attention to your food and savour its flavours and textures, so that when you

FAT FALLACY

GRAZING CAN HELP YOU LOSE WEIGHT

It is a myth that eating little and often can help you to lose weight. What matters is the total number of calories you consume in a day. If you spread your calorie intake over the day you will have more energy and more stable blood sugar levels, but you must also reduce the number of calories you consume each day if you want to lose weight.

have finished it you will feel satisfied.

Give yourself at least twenty minutes for your meal – your brain's appetite centre remains switched on for about twenty minutes each time you eat, so within that time is the 'danger zone' in which you are more likely to want food again. This is also the length of time it usually takes for the satiety signals that register the feeling of fullness to reach your appetite centre.

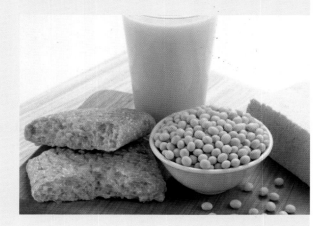

5 STICK TO DIETARY GUIDELINES

Follow the dietary guidelines (see pages 133–9) and make sure your meals contain foods such as beans, pulses and whole-grain bread that are likely to help control your appetite. If you choose sugary, low-fibre foods they will give you a short energy burst but leave you hungry soon after, and then you will find it difficult to keep to planned meal times and will soon be reaching for a snack.

PRACTICAL TIPS

If you occasionally find it difficult to stick to specific meal times, then at least graze on healthy snacks such as fruit and vegetables.

• Try not to buy high-calorie, poor-quality snack foods in the first place, not even for the children. There is a lot of pressure on parents to buy such foods, but if you resist you will be doing a great service for your children as well as for yourself. Why not involve the children in cooking some healthier snacks at home together?

• Resist the temptation to eat leftover food. Many people find it morally objectionable to throw food away, so ideally either get into the habit of cooking less to begin with or cook enough so that you can keep some for another meal. Otherwise, remind yourself that discarding it is still better than compromising your own health.

• Brush your teeth immediately after each meal, to reinforce the idea that you have finished eating.

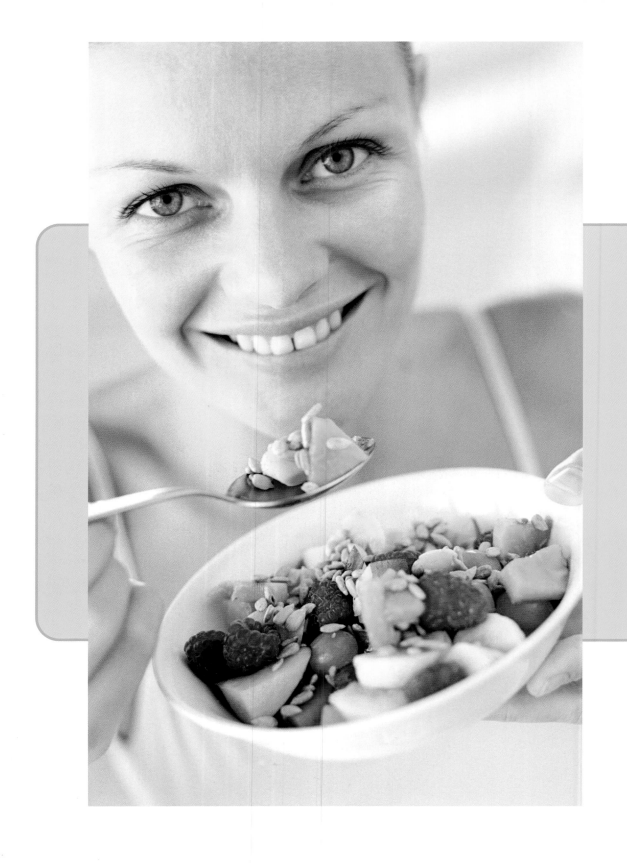

2

APPETITE AND DIGESTION

APPETITE AND HUNGER

Your body is constantly using up energy, even when you're asleep, and it gets this energy from the 'fuels' that it makes from your food (see page 51). These fuels circulate in your bloodstream and your body has a well-developed system – like an inbuilt fuel gauge – that monitors their levels. Whenever supplies are running low, this system triggers feelings of hunger that prompt you to eat again and restore your energy levels. It ultimately controls how often you eat and how much you eat each time, and so it also controls your total daily calorie intake.

This eating control system is based on four main sensory signals: hunger, satiation, satiety and appetite. Hunger is the uncomfortable feeling that drives you to eat, while satiation is the feeling of fullness that tells you when to stop eating. Satiety follows satiation, and is the feeling of being replete that dispels hunger until your energy levels start to drop again and you are ready for your next meal. Appetite is your desire to eat, especially to eat specific foods. It is not the same as hunger – the need to eat – and is not an uncomfortable feeling.

Although appetite is a desire rather than a need, hunger, satiation and satiety all have some influence on it. They are generated in the appetite centre of your brain, in response to signals from your body about the amount of food you have eaten and the levels of circulating fuel. They combine to either stimulate or suppress your appetite, and affect your food intake over a period of several hours, between meals. Another set of sensory signals, based on the sight, smell, taste and texture of your food, have a more immediate effect on your appetite and food intake and come into play while you are actually eating.

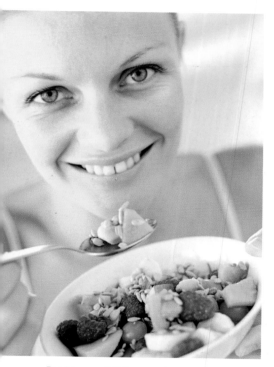

Food is one of life's great pleasures, and most healthy people have a good appetite, so that their needs for 'fuel' are met.

KNOWING WHEN TO STOP

To extract energy from food, your body has to first break it down (digest it), then separate and absorb the valuable nutrients before eliminating the waste. Digestion begins in your mouth, with chewing, and continues in your stomach and intestines with the help of acid and enzymes, proteins that speed up biochemical reactions. Eating food that has bulk will stretch the walls of your stomach, which is normally about the size of a grapefruit, and this stretching

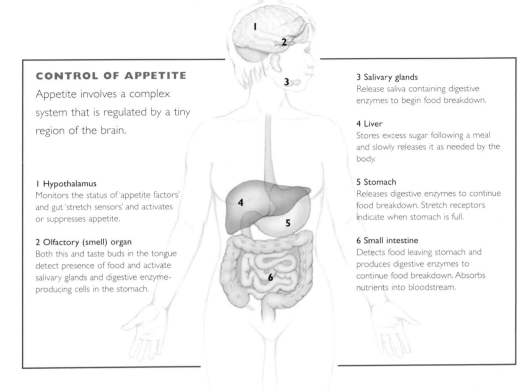

CONTROL OF APPETITE

Appetite involves a complex system that is regulated by a tiny region of the brain.

1 Hypothalamus
Monitors the status of 'appetite factors' and gut 'stretch sensors' and activates or suppresses appetite.

2 Olfactory (smell) organ
Both this and taste buds in the tongue detect presence of food and activate salivary glands and digestive enzyme-producing cells in the stomach.

3 Salivary glands
Release saliva containing digestive enzymes to begin food breakdown.

4 Liver
Stores excess sugar following a meal and slowly releases it as needed by the body.

5 Stomach
Releases digestive enzymes to continue food breakdown. Stretch receptors indicate when stomach is full.

6 Small intestine
Detects food leaving stomach and produces digestive enzymes to continue food breakdown. Absorbs nutrients into bloodstream.

sends signals to your brain and triggers the feeling of satiation, which eventually stops you from eating. The longer the food takes to digest, the longer it will stay in your stomach and the longer you will feel full.

The 'stretch point' at which your stomach triggers satiation may be partly genetic, but regularly taking in large volumes of food or drink can overstretch it so that you need more food before you feel full. It is possible, however, to reset this stretch point by eating smaller volumes of food, enabling your stomach to shrink back to its normal size and regain its sensitivity.

GETTING HUNGRY AGAIN

After digestion, energy-rich nutrients such as fats and glucose are absorbed from your small intestine into your bloodstream, which delivers them to your body cells for use as fuel. Satiety and hunger are both intimately linked to the levels of glucose in your circulation (your blood sugar levels). When your blood sugar is above a certain level you feel sated, and when it falls you will experience cravings and then hunger, so regulating your blood sugar is the key to controlling your appetite.

The longer your food can maintain your blood sugar levels, the longer it will dispel hunger, and this is related to the speed at which the food is digested. Sugary foods, for example, are quickly digested and give your blood sugar levels a rapid boost, but their effects are short-lived and you soon feel hungry again. Whole grain starchy foods, such as porridge oats and brown rice, take longer to digest and release their energy more gradually, so they stave off the hunger pangs for much longer.

SATISFACTION

The feeling of satisfaction that you get after a meal is more complex because it combines the feelings of satiation and satiety together with the overall sensory experience of eating. For instance, you can drink a litre of water and feel full but not satisfied, and you can sustain yourself on teaspoonfuls of sugar so that you do not feel hungry but again, you will not feel full or satisfied. The feeling of satisfaction is difficult to define biologically, but most people know it instinctively.

SATISFYING YOUR APPETITE

Hunger, satiation, satiety and the food you eat are not the only factors that influence your appetite. Appetite is also affected by metabolic changes in your body, such as those brought on by injury or stress, and by your natural sleep/wake cycles. Additionally, such factors as your moods and emotions, the sensory appeal of food, your environment and your social circumstances will all affect how hungry you feel.

However, by choosing foods that are more likely to make you feel full and keep you sated for longer, it is possible to satisfy your appetite and reduce your calorie

THE FOOD PYRAMID

Devised by the US Department of Agriculture (USDA), is a visual image that illustrates how much of each type of food you should eat each day to achieve a healthy diet. The pyramid has four levels, with whole grains and cereals making up the large base. Vegetables and fruits make up the next level, followed by meat and milk products as the third level and fats, oils and sweets making up the small tip of the pyramid.

Build up your daily diet in the same way. Eat lots of whole grains, cereals, rice and pasta, plenty of vegetables and fruits, two or three servings each of meat and milk products, and sparing amounts of additional fats, oils and sweeteners.

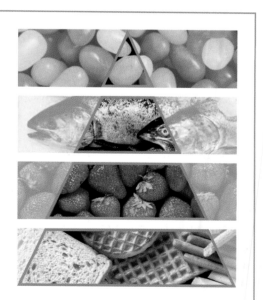

intake at the same time in order to lose weight. Choosing foods that will automatically help you to regulate your appetite is at the heart of long-term weight management.

One factor to bear in mind, though, is that appetite control is asymmetrical. In other words, the biological drive to overeat is much greater than the drive to under-eat. Under-eating increases your desire to eat, but so does overeating, and deliberate under-eating is more uncomfortable than overeating.

ENERGY FROM FOOD

The energy in food comes from four main sources – carbohydrate, protein, fat and alcohol – and foods may contain any or all of these in different combinations and quantities. Your body, however, uses each of them in a different way. For example, although fat is the most energy-dense component of food (see pages 60–62), your body prefers not to use it immediately if others, especially carbohydrates, are available. In fact, in a mixed meal, the energy-providing constituents of the food are used in the following order:

1. **Alcohol:** your body cannot store alcohol so it has to use it for fuel immediately
2. **Carbohydrate:** this is your body's preferred source of fuel
3. **Protein:** ideally reserved for building and maintaining your body tissues
4. **Fat:** the last component to be used for fuel.

So if you eat a mixed meal, your body will use alcohol for energy first, then carbohydrate, then protein, and then if it still needs more energy it will use the fat. Naturally, there is great individual variation so some people are better able to use fat for energy, but essentially all of these energy sources can be used for fuel and excess calories from any of them can be converted to body fat.

CARBOHYDRATES

Carbohydrates are the sugars and starches from which your body makes most of its energy-providing glucose, and their main sources are fruits, vegetables and whole grains. The sugars in foods include glucose, fructose (fruit sugar), galactose and sucrose (cane or beet sugar), while long chains of glucose molecules make up the starches, which plants produce as a way of storing glucose as an energy reserve.

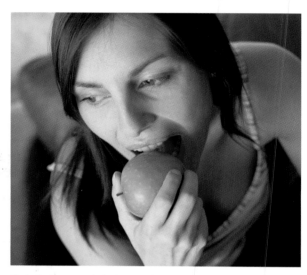

Carbohydrates get 'a bad press' from time to time, but good sources are essential to your health. Fruits, vegetables, seeds and grains are necessary for your body's energy needs.

Another type of glucose chain, cellulose, is one of the main structural materials of plants. Although the human body can't digest cellulose, it is a valuable part of a healthy diet because it's an important constituent of dietary fibre, which adds bulk to meals and makes them filling without itself being fattening.

The carbohydrates that you can digest are broken down in your mouth, stomach and intestines into the basic sugars glucose, fructose and galactose, which are then absorbed into your bloodstream. The glucose is immediately available as an energy source, but the fructose and galactose must first pass through your liver, where they are converted into glucose before re-entering your bloodstream.

The amount of glucose which, at any one time, circulates in your bloodstream is referred to as your blood glucose or blood sugar level, and this rises as you digest and absorb the carbohydrates in your food. However, your body has to stop your blood sugar levels from rising too far, because excessive blood sugar can, over time, damage your brain and other vital organs.

CONTROLLING BLOOD SUGAR

If your blood sugar level starts to rise too high after you've eaten, your pancreas releases the hormone insulin into your bloodstream. Insulin lowers your blood sugar level by stimulating your muscles, fat cells and various organs (especially your liver) to remove glucose from your bloodstream.

The insulin encourages your muscle cells and other body cells to use the glucose for fuel, rather than using fat or protein, so at the same time it stops you from using

TO LOSE WEIGHT YOU HAVE TO GO HUNGRY

In fact, when your blood sugar is low, your body will burn muscle and fat but will also slow down your metabolism, which can stop you from losing weight. If you eat the right foods, you can lose weight and satisfy your appetite without disturbing your metabolism.

your fat reserves. It also prompts your muscles and liver to convert some of the excess glucose into glycogen and store it as an energy reserve, and your fat cells to take up the remainder and convert it into body fat. Then, as your blood sugar level falls, so does the level of insulin secretion.

The amount of insulin that your body secretes over the course of a day depends on the types of carbohydrate that you eat, and can affect your appetite as well as your ability to burn fat. When you eat 'fast-release' carbohydrates – those that are that are digested quickly, such as sugary snacks – they pass rapidly through your stomach and so they don't keep you full. They also cause a fast release of glucose into your bloodstream, so your blood sugar rises quickly, initially making you feel satisfied, highly energized or even, a little 'high'.

The rapid rise in your blood sugar also stimulates an equally rapid release of large amounts of insulin. This flood of insulin produces a sudden fall in your blood sugar, at which point you may experience fatigue, drowsiness, inability to concentrate, light-headedness, headaches or irritability.

The fall in blood sugar can also bring cravings for another snack or sugar hit. This is because your body prefers to hang on to its stored fat rather than convert it into the blood sugar it needs, so it tries to drive you towards consumption by generating uncomfortable feelings such as cravings or hunger. These rapid swings in blood sugar and insulin secretion result in highs and lows of mood and energy, and cravings that are more likely to increase your calorie intake over the day with the excess sugar being converted into body fat.

In contrast, 'slow-release' carbohydrates, such as whole-grain bread, are digested slowly and will remain in your stomach for longer, keeping you fuller for longer and release

STRESS AND BLOOD SUGAR LEVELS

When you eat a lot of sugary foods, you become caught in a vicious circle. The sugary foods provide you with an initial lift that quickly turns into a downer making you crave further sugary foods.

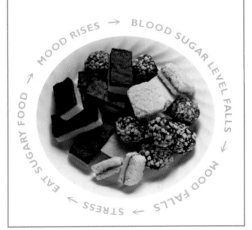

MOOD RISES → BLOOD SUGAR LEVEL FALLS ↘ MOOD FALLS ← STRESS → EAT SUGARY FOOD ↗

glucose into your bloodstream more slowly. They produce a much more gradual rise in your blood sugar so they also stimulate a much smaller rise in insulin secretion. Their overall effect is to provide your body with a steady supply of energy, while keeping your blood sugar level stable and so avoiding rapid swings in your mood and energy. They maintain satiety and reduce cravings and hunger, which helps you to control your appetite. Less insulin in your bloodstream also allows your body to access its fat reserves, making weight loss easier and more comfortable.

So how do you differentiate between fast-release and slow-release carbohydrate foods? There are two properties to look for: the amount of dietary fibre in the food and the degree of processing and refinement it has undergone. The more fibre it has and the less processed it is, the more likely it is to be high in slow-release carbohydrates.

FILLING FIBRE

The presence of dietary fibre in a food is, however, more than just a sign that it contains slow-release carbohydrates. Dietary fibre is itself good for your health and it also helps you to control your food intake. It cannot be digested, has no energy content and is left over after the digestible carbohydrates have been absorbed by your small intestine. It then passes into your large intestine where it is partly broken down by bacteria (a process that unfortunately produces gas) but absorbs excess water and adds bulk to your stools.

Fibre helps you to reduce your intake of food in a number of useful ways. For example, it gives food a more substantial texture so that it takes

FIBRE CONTENT OF COMMON FOODS PER 100 GRAMS

WHOLE-GRAIN FLOUR	9
WHOLE-GRAIN BREAD	6
BROWN RICE	1
CORN FLAKES	1
ALMONDS	7
BRAZIL NUTS	4
HAZELNUTS	7
PEANUTS	6
WALNUTS	3.5
APPLES	2
AVOCADOS	3.5
CARROTS	2.5
LEEKS	2
SPINACH	2
CABBAGE	2
SWEET CORN	1
LIMA BEANS	7
BAKED BEANS (CANNED)	4
GREEN BEANS	6
PEAS	5
APRICOTS	6
PRUNES	6
DATES	5
RAISINS	2

- CEREALS AND RICE
- FRUIT AND VEGETABLES
- DRIED FRUIT
- NUTS
- PEAS AND BEANS

longer to chew and thus to reach your stomach – food that lacks fibre has a melt-in-the-mouth quality and is rapidly chewed. Fibre also provides bulk, so once it reaches your stomach it helps to fill you up.

In your small intestine, fibre in foods makes it harder for your digestive enzymes to break them down, so digestion takes longer. To prevent itself from becoming overloaded, your small intestine then releases a hormone called cholecystokinin, which slows down the rate at which your stomach empties. This keeps your stomach distended for longer and you feeling fuller. The release of cholecystokinin usually takes about 20 minutes, so eating more slowly will help time the sensation of feeling full to coincide with the end of your meal.

Foods that are high in natural fibre are generally slow-release carbohydrates, and studies indicate that eating an additional 14 grams of fibre per day for more than three days is associated with a 10 percent reduction in calorie intake. Carbohydrates that lack fibre, or have had the fibre removed, are mostly fast-release so they don't keep you full for long or maintain satiety. It is easy to eat significant amounts and still become hungry a short time later. Be sure to choose your sources of fibre carefully as some – such as nuts and seeds – are also high in calories.

DON'T EAT WHEN YOU'RE NOT HUNGRY

If you eat when you are not remotely hungry, you are taking in energy at a time when your blood sugar is already high so what you eat is more likely to be converted into body fat.

PROCESSED FOODS

Foods that are processed or refined in any way before you eat them are easier to chew and digest than fibre-rich whole foods, so their nutrients are absorbed more quickly and reach your bloodstream sooner. They are less likely to remain in your intestines and keep you feeling full, and less able to maintain satiety. Essentially, processing and refinement changes the structure of the food, turning a slow-release carbohydrate into a fast-release. This is especially true of refined, energy-dense carbohydrates that have been stripped of their natural structure and fibre.

Processing includes not only the industrial processing and refining of raw materials, such as flour and sugar, but also some methods of preparing food before you eat it. These include prolonged cooking, chopping, puréeing, liquefying and juicing, all of which break down or remove the fibre. This can ease digestion but is less good for controlling appetite.

The speed at which digestion and absorption occurs also depends on the inner structure of the carbohydrate, which can affect its classification as a fast-release or slow-release carbohydrate. To make it easier to differentiate between the two, dietitians have created the concept of the glycaemic index.

THE GLYCAEMIC INDEX

The glycaemic index (GI) is a crude measure of how rapidly a carbohydrate food is digested and absorbed from your small intestine, and how quickly it raises your blood glucose and triggers insulin release. The GI value of a food is calculated by feeding people a portion of it containing 50 grams of carbohydrate, then measuring the subsequent rise in their blood glucose.

The index uses a 50-gram dose of pure glucose, which has a GI value of 100, as the standard, so eating foods that have a GI value close to 100 will raise your blood sugar as rapidly as eating pure glucose will – very rapidly indeed. Foods with lower GI values will have less impact on your blood sugar levels. Those that have a GI value of less than 55 are slow-release carbohydrates that raise blood sugar levels slowly, whereas those with a GI value greater than 55 are fast-release.

On the whole, foods containing complex, high-fibre unrefined carbohydrates have lower GI values than those containing large amounts of refined carbohydrates and simple sugars. Low-GI foods tend to be more filling and help you to maintain stable blood sugar levels, while high-GI foods tend to stimulate excessive insulin production. This causes rapid swings in your blood sugar levels, triggering cravings and reducing your energy.

The GI is useful as a guide, but it has limitations that you must keep in mind when using it to choose between foods. Firstly, the index tells you nothing about calories or nutrition. A low GI does not mean low calorie. For instance, a Mars bar has a lower GI than a banana but has more calories and less nutritional value, so remember that calories still count!

FAT FACT

LOW GI IS BETTER THAN LOW CALORIES

Studies have found that individuals who were allowed to eat as much as they want lose more weight by eating low-GI foods than by sticking to a calorie-controlled, low-fat diet.

HIGH-GLYCAEMIC-INDEX FOODS (GI GREATER THAN 50)

Glucose	Doughnuts	Crisps
Honey	Crispbread	Melon
Refined sugar	Bagels	Mango
Muesli	Rice cakes	Banana
Whole-wheat cereals	Rice	Pumpkin
Cornflakes	Biscuits	Pineapple
White bread	Parsnips	Chocolates/sweets
French bread	Potatoes	Ice cream
Waffles	Chips	Soft drinks

Secondly, the GI does not measure portion size in weight: a GI portion is one that contains 50 grams of carbohydrate, but the portion itself may weigh much more. Watermelon, for example, has a higher GI than raisins, but you would need to eat a very large portion of it to get the same amount of carbohydrate that you would get from a small helping of raisins. And charts and lists of GI values often do not include common vegetables such as lettuce, cabbage and celery, because it would take a very large portion of these to supply 50 grams of digestible

carbohydrate, much more than is humanly possible to eat in one serving. You can eat as much of these vegetables as you want without worrying about their effect on your blood sugar levels.

Thirdly, the components of a mixed meal interact with each other and alter its overall GI in a possibly misleading way. Fat, for example, can reduce the GI of a meal, but it also increases its calorie content.

Finally, the GIs of foods are measured under strict laboratory conditions involving small samples of people who have been fasting to standardize their blood sugar levels. This is unlike normal conditions, where people's blood sugar levels are affected by exercise, dehydration, stomach acidity, length of time between meals, stress, smoking, alcohol, and some spices and/or medications. In other words, the science here is not precise and GI values should be used only as a general guide.

LOW-GLYCAEMIC-INDEX FOODS (GI LESS THAN 50)

Fructose	Yogurt	Most beans
Grapes	Nuts	(including
Oranges	Pasta	baked beans)
Apples	Whole grain bread	
Pears	Oats	
Cherries	Bran	
Fruit juice	Most vegetables (such as carrots,	
Apricots (fresh and dried)	tomatoes, broccoli, watercress	
Milk	courgettes)	

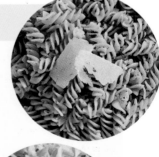
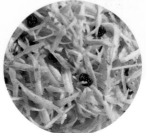

PROTEINS

Proteins are essential constituents of the bodies of all living creatures, and in the human body they help to form the structure of body cells and tissues such as muscle, skin and bone. You can get the proteins you need from many types of food, including meat, dairy products, cereals, nuts, beans and soya products.

Proteins are made up of long chains of smaller molecules called amino acids. When you eat proteins, your body does not use them directly to build and repair its own tissues, Instead, your digestive system breaks them down into their component amino acids, and your body then reassembles these amino acids in different ways to make the particular proteins that it needs.

Because all cells need protein for building their structures and to assist their general functioning, your body prefers to use its dietary protein for these purposes. However, your body can use protein to produce energy if necessary – even protein from its own muscle tissue – and it can also convert spare dietary protein into body fat.

PROTEINS AND ESSENTIAL AMINO ACIDS

The human body contains more than 10,000 different proteins, assembled from different combinations of about 22 amino acids. Eight of these amino acids – isoleucine, leucine, lysine, methionine, phenylalanine, threonine, tryptophan and valine – are classified as 'essential amino acids' because your body cannot make them itself and so it must get them from proteins in your food. Two other amino acids, arginine and histidine, are essential in children but not in adults. In general, proteins from meat, fish, eggs and soya contain all the essential amino acids, but proteins from other foods will lack one or more of them and be 'incomplete'. Vegetarians, therefore, should make sure they get their protein from a wide selection of different cereals, beans, lentils, seeds and nuts.

DIGESTING PROTEINS

The digestion of dietary protein is not unlike that of carbohydrates, but it is amino acids not sugars that are released and absorbed into your bloodstream. Your bloodstream carries the amino acids to your liver, where they either continue to circulate in the blood to be picked up by cells as needed, or are converted into glucose and used to maintain your blood sugar levels and supply energy. Any not needed for these purposes can be converted to body fat.

Protein has a favourable effect on your appetite because it is digested very slowly. Most sources of protein have a substantial texture and need plenty of chewing, and in the stomach their bulk can help to fill you up. Protein also triggers the release of cholecystokinin (see page 55), which slows down stomach emptying and so keeps you feeling fuller for longer.

After absorption, the conversion of amino acids to glucose to supply energy occurs at a stable pace and releases a steady flow of glucose into your bloodstream, which maintains satiety. Some insulin is released, but so are counteractive hormones such as glucagon, which mostly cancel out its effects so that a sudden fall in your blood sugar level is avoided.

PROTEIN AND CARBOHYDRATE

Most dietary protein sources such as meat, cheese and eggs have an effect on blood sugar equivalent to a carbohydrate with a GI value of between 30 and 40. However, you should not use protein (especially animal protein) instead of slow-release carbohydrates as a dietary source of energy, despite its ability to suppress appetite. Eating too much protein puts stress on your liver and kidneys, and excessive consumption of animal protein is associated with increased risks of cancer and heart disease. You will also miss out on the nutritional benefits of the dietary fibre, vitamins, minerals and antioxidants usually found in natural high-fibre carbohydrate foods.

Your body functions best with carbohydrate as its fuel, reserving protein for cell building and maintenance. In terms of controlling appetite and promoting health, moderate amounts of lean, good-quality sources of protein can make a valuable contribution to your diet when combined with slow-release carbohydrates.

QUALITY OF PROTEIN IN FOOD

A food's protein quality is determined by the amounts of essential amino acids that it contains. Eggs are the most complete protein – they have a maximum score of 100. This chart shows the protein quality of foods as measured against the egg.

Protein source	Protein quality
Egg	100
Fish	90
Meat	80
Cow's milk	80
Grain with pulses (peas or lentils)	80
Soya beans	75
Oatmeal	65
Rice	57
Peas	48
Lentils	45
Kidney beans	44
Whole grain bread	40

FATS

Fats, also referred to as lipids, play many important roles in the human body. As well as being the body's main energy store, they are vital components of cell structures and of many hormones and other biologically active substances. In addition, a number of essential vitamins (A, D, E and K) can only be absorbed by your small intestine if they are first dissolved in fat, so you need some fat in your diet to enable this to happen.

Depending on its source, dietary fat consists of either triglycerides or cholesterol, or of a combination of the two. Triglycerides are present in both plants and animals and are a potential source of fuel, while cholesterol is found in all animal food products but is virtually absent from plants. In the body, dietary cholesterol is not used as fuel but it has many other, other important functions.

DIGESTING FAT

Your body takes a long time to digest fat, a process that occurs mostly in your small intestine and involves enzymes and bile. Bile, a substance that your liver makes from cholesterol, is stored in your gallbladder and helps to dissolve fat in water.

After digestion is complete, free fatty acids (fatty acids that are no longer in triglyceride chains), glycerol and cholesterol are released and enter your bloodstream. When they reach your liver, they are either returned to your bloodstream to be used as fuel or they are sent to body fat stores. The bile is recycled by your liver to be used again.

FAT AS FOOD

When you eat fat by itself, it is not very filling because it lacks bulk. But fat is a potent stimulator of cholecystokinin, which slows down the rate at which your stomach empties, so if you eat it together with foods that have bulk, such as high-fibre carbohydrates and/or protein, it can help to keep you feeling fuller for longer. Similarly, fat on its own has no effect on your blood sugar or insulin levels, but in a mixed meal it can lower the overall glycaemic index and so increase satiety.

Both of these factors may help you to reduce your calorie intake but only up to a point, after which increasing fat does not continue to increase satiety. In studies, the effect on appetite was the same with meals that contained 10, 20 and 40 percent fat.

DIETARY FATS IN COMMON COOKING OILS

This chart shows the proportions of saturated, monounsaturated and polyunsaturated fatty acids in various cooking fats. Also shown are the levels of linoleic and linolenic essential fatty acids, which are found in polyunsaturated fat.

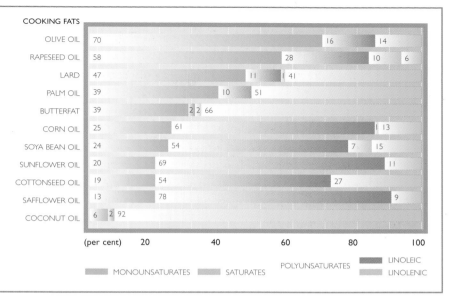

COOKING FATS

OLIVE OIL	70	16	14	
RAPESEED OIL	58	28	10	6
LARD	47	11	41	
PALM OIL	39	10	51	
BUTTERFAT	39	2 2 66		
CORN OIL	25	61	1 13	
SOYA BEAN OIL	24	54	7	15
SUNFLOWER OIL	20	69	11	
COTTONSEED OIL	19	54	27	
SAFFLOWER OIL	13	78	9	
COCONUT OIL	6 2 92			

(per cent) 20 40 60 80 100

MONOUNSATURATES   SATURATES   POLYUNSATURATES   LINOLEIC   LINOLENIC

SATURATED OR UNSATURATED FATS

Fats are classified as either saturated or unsaturated. A saturated fat has two hydrogen atoms attached to each carbon atom. There is no room for any more hydrogen, so the fat is 'saturated'. An unsaturated fat is missing some hydrogen atoms – a monounsaturated fat lacks a pair of hydrogen atoms, a polyunsaturated fat may lack two or more pairs.

Saturated fats are normally solid at room temperature. Unsaturated fats are usually liquid but can be made solid by adding hydrogen atoms to them, turning them into 'trans fatty acids', or 'transfats'. These are often used in manufactured foods such as margarines, and are thought to be potentially harmful because when eaten they increase harmful LDL cholesterol in the bloodstream and lower beneficial HDL cholesterol.

Fat is also very energy-dense, so increasing the fat content of a meal above 10 percent will do nothing to increase satiety but will add considerably to your calorie intake. This is especially true if the fat is combined with simple refined carbohydrates that lack fibre and bulk; these foods will not fill you up and the taste combination can actually increase your appetite.

Your body can use dietary fat as a fuel by converting it in your liver into glucose or into ketones (substances that it can use in place of glucose), but it will do this only as a last resort. This 'fat-sparing' effect means that fat in a mixed meal is more readily stored as body fat, because carbohydrates and proteins in your food have to be converted into fat whereas dietary fat comes ready for storage. There is a fine line between having just enough fat in your diet to control appetite and satisfy taste, and too much fat that can increase calorie intake.

FATS AND HEALTH

In terms of overall health, excessive intake of some forms of dietary fat has been associated with a number of serious diseases that are linked to high levels of lipids in the blood. When blood is tested for levels of lipids, what is usually measured is the amounts of total cholesterol, LDL cholesterol, HDL cholesterol and triglycerides.

Fat is not soluble in blood, so it is transported in your bloodstream by proteins called lipoproteins. LDL (low-density lipoprotein) cholesterol carries fat from your liver to your body tissues and is associated with the build-up of fat deposits (fatty plaques) that block arteries and can cause heart disease. HDL (high-density lipoprotein) cholesterol, however, actually removes excess cholesterol from your circulation and takes it back to your liver, which converts it into bile.

ESSENTIAL FATTY ACIDS

As with amino acids (see page 58), there are some fatty acids that the body needs but is unable to make for itself. These 'essential fatty acids' are linoleic acid (one of the 'omega 6' family of fatty acids) and alpha-linolenic acid (an 'omega 3' fatty acid). Good dietary sources of these fatty acids include vegetable oils and leafy green vegetables.

The level of LDL-cholesterol in your blood is affected by the rate at which your liver removes it, which is partly genetic. However, there is also a strong link between excessive consumption of saturated fats and transfats (see box), raised levels of total and LDL-cholesterol and/or triglycerides, and an increased risk of heart disease. These three are the harmful, unhealthy blood fats, and you can help to reduce them by cutting down on saturated fat and increasing dietary fibre and exercise. Raised levels of HDL-cholesterol appear to protect against heart disease by removing fatty deposits, and you can boost levels of this 'healthy' fat by increasing physical activity and your intake of unsaturated fats and natural fibre.

So exactly how much fat should you include in your diet? Fat is used very efficiently in your body, so even when you are on a very-low-fat diet there is little danger of becoming deficient in it. Ideally, your fat consumption should consist of small amounts of unsaturated fats together with slow-release carbohydrates and protein. This will be enough to satisfy your appetite without adding too many calories.

FAT FACT

A HIGH-FAT DIET AIDS DIGESTION

A high-fat diet makes your body better at digesting fats so the ability of fat to limit your food intake by increasing satiation and satiety is gradually reduced. This may be a factor that makes it difficult for obese people to lose weight.

ALCOHOL

Alcohol is absorbed directly into your bloodstream from your stomach and small intestine. As it has no bulk, it will not make you feel full, although alcoholic drinks such as beer and lager, which are taken in large volumes, can expand in your stomach and fill you up – but only for while. In the long term, these drinks can actually stretch your stomach (hence the term 'beer belly'), which is counterproductive.

Alcohol provides energy but it has no satiety value, and too much actually lowers your blood sugar and dehydrates you, making you hungry. It also stimulates your appetite directly because it enters your brain, where it lowers your inhibitions in general and disinhibits your appetite in the process. This lowering of inhibitions also affects your senses, emotions, reasoning and thoughts and so it can weaken your resolve, making you more likely to overeat or even binge.

Eating food with alcohol will delay its absorption and so dampen some of these effects, but this only increases your calorie intake and many alcoholic cocktails, such as cream liqueurs, are already very high in fat and sugar.

Despite these drawbacks, research has confirmed that moderate consumption of antioxidant-rich red wine, can be beneficial by reducing high blood fats, high blood pressure, heart disease and strokes. However, it is possible to derive these benefits by other means, such as eating a healthy diet and taking plenty of exercise.

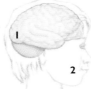

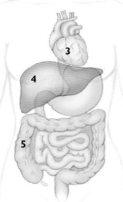

THE PERILS OF EXCESSIVE DRINKING

Imbibing high levels of alcohol can have a number of potentially serious side effects.

1 Depression
Heavy alcohol consumption gradually destroys the brain cells, and can result in depression, memory loss and intellectual deterioration.

2 Mouth and throat cancer
High levels of alcohol intake increase the risk of cancers of the mouth, tongue and throat.

3 Heart disease
Heavy drinkers are more susceptible to coronary heart disease and hypertension (high blood pressure) and are more likely to suffer a stroke.

4 Liver disease
Persistent and excessive consumption may lead to fatty liver, alcoholic hepatitis, cirrhosis and liver cancer.

5 Digestive disorders
Heavy drinkers may suffer from digestive tract diseases, such as gastritis, pancreatitis and cancer of the upper digestive tract.

6 Nerve damage
Malnutrition, common among alcoholics, disturbs nerve functioning, causing symptoms such as cramps and numbness.

INSATIABLE APPETITE

Some people find that no matter how much they eat, they seem to feel hungry all the time. This leads them to eat too much at each meal, and to fill in the gaps between meals with frequent snacks. The inevitable result is that every day they take in far more calories than they need, and their weight relentlessly increases.

CASE HISTORY

MARIA'S weight had increased steadily over the past few years, despite her repeated attempts to control it. Every time she tried to lose some by cutting back on her food intake, she would find she was hungry all the time and so would give up. She claimed that her problem food was bread, and her food diary seemed to support this admission. White bread, in various guises including French baguettes, muffins and pitta bread, featured consistently in her meals, especially breakfast and lunch. What also emerged from the diary was her regular snacking on tea and biscuits throughout the day, in addition to her meals, either because she was hungry or lacked energy. She had a full-time, office-based job that did not involve much physical activity, so her average calorie intake was well in excess of her needs, which accounted for her gradual weight gain.

WHAT CAUSES IT?

To understand why you may feel hungry soon after a large meal, you have to go back to some basic principles of physiology. True hunger is a signal that is related to the amount of glucose circulating in your bloodstream. When your haven't eaten for a while, your blood sugar levels fall. Then you experience cravings or hunger, which are your body's way of prompting you to eat so that your blood sugar levels rise again. So, it is natural to feel hungry if you haven't eaten for a long time, but why do you feel hungry soon after a substantial meal? One reason is that you've been eating the wrong foods.

When you eat, the food enters your stomach and intestines where it is digested and absorbed into your bloodstream, so raising your blood sugar levels. Some foods, especially refined, starchy carbohydrates, are quickly digested and the nutrients that they contain, such as glucose and amino acids, are absorbed into your bloodstream equally quickly.

The speed at which this happens generally depends on how much processing the food has undergone before you eat it, and the amount of natural fibre it contains. For example, food that is made with refined ingredients such as white flour and sugar, and has had most of its natural fibre removed, lacks bulk so you have to eat more of it to feel full. You will also digest it very quickly, so eating it leads to a rapid rise in your blood sugar. Such foods are said to have a high glycaemic index (GI, see pages 56–7). Foods that are made with less-refined ingredients (such as whole grains) make you feel fuller sooner and produce much slower rises in your blood sugar, and have a low glycaemic index and keep you fuller for longer.

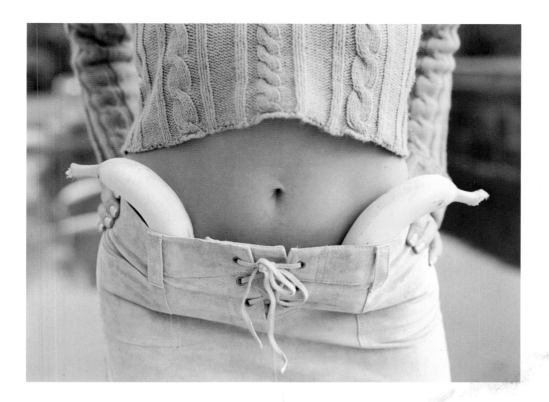

Having a high blood sugar level might seem to be a good thing because it stops you from feeling hungry, but it turns out that blood sugar appears to follow the old adage: the faster the rise, the harder the fall. When you eat food that raises your blood sugar rapidly, your body reacts by releasing large amounts of insulin into your bloodstream to prevent your blood sugar from becoming dangerously high (see pages 56–7). This can actually cause a rapid fall in your blood sugar levels a short time later. The amount of insulin released is closely related to the rate at which your blood sugar rises – faster it rises, the more insulin is secreted and so the faster it falls.

When hunger strikes, it's important to reach for something to eat that will keep your blood sugar levels from rising too high.

THE CONSEQUENCES

So what does the relationship between insulin and the glycaemic index mean for you when you are trying to lose weight? Eating food with a high GI, such as white bread, makes you feel sated for a short time, but it triggers the release of large amounts of insulin, so your blood sugar level rapidly drops back and you soon feel hungry again. Trying to control your appetite and food intake when you regularly eat high-GI foods is very difficult indeed because you are constantly battling against hunger and cravings, powerful drives that are difficult to resist with sheer willpower. If a large

HIDDEN SUGAR

You should be aware of the hidden sugar content of many processed foods. Economy brands, in particular, are likely to contain added sugar as it provides taste, but even so-called 'health' bars – sold as healthy, low-fat snacks – can be packed with sugar (and processed fats). Always read the label and look out for ingredients such as dextrose, sucrose, fructose, corn syrup, malt and sorbitol – these are all sugars by another name.

part of your diet consists of high-GI foods, you are very likely to eat more and thus gain weight.

Foods with lower GIs, however, trigger smaller amounts of insulin and so your blood sugar remains more stable and falls more slowly, preventing hunger for longer. When you eat foods with a low GI, you will find it easier to control both your appetite and your weight.

Your blood sugar levels also have an effect on your energy levels and moods, because glucose is the body's preferred source of fuel and the one that the brain works best with. When you eat food that generates a rapid rise in blood sugar, you may experience an initial burst of energy and a sugar 'buzz'. But that will soon fade, leaving you lethargic, tired, and lacking in concentration, and possibly irritable and short-tempered. If you then reach for a sugary, high-GI snack, the process will start all over again as your blood sugar level, energy and mood continue on this roller-coaster ride together.

And what happens to all the extra sugar in your bloodstream when you eat high-GI foods? Unfortunately, the insulin released to control it also puts your body into fat-storage mode, the excess sugar is channelled away from your bloodstream and converted into body fat. In other words, because all the calories you are eating arrive at the same time, instead of in a steady flow, your body is unable to use all of them immediately so it stores some as body fat.

Maria (see page 64) was constantly fighting a losing battle against precisely these forces every day. She was taking in a large number of calories, but because her body was processing them very quickly, she would feel satisfied for only a short time before hunger and cravings struck her again.

Her initial response would be to resist, but she couldn't hold out for very long. She would inevitably reach for a snack to dispel her hunger and sustain her energy levels and concentration, even though its effects were short-lived. Although Maria's problem was with white bread and other refined carbohydrate foods, the basic principles apply to foods in general. The faster your body assimilates the energy from any food, the sooner it will demand more by triggering hunger and cravings.

Insatiable Appetite Recovery Program

1 FIND THE CAUSE

First of all, you must be clear that the hunger you are experiencing is genuinely physical hunger. For example, it may be that your urge to eat is actually driven by emotional hunger arising from stress, anxiety, or other uncomfortable feelings, and you are using food as a coping mechanism. Sometimes, it can be hard to tell the difference between emotional hunger and physical hunger, so if you are unsure, keep a food and mood diary for a week or so and look for any patterns of eating that relate to emotionally stressful situations (see pages 91–2).

FAT FALLACY

TOO MUCH CARBOHYDRATE MAKES YOU FAT

This is not true. It is too many calories, whether they are from carbohydrates, fat or protein that makes you fat. The trick is to eat the right carbohydrates – those that keep you full so that you eat fewer calories.

Other causes of low blood sugar and hunger include high-intensity aerobic exercise – which uses up all your blood sugar to fuel your muscles – and some stimulants, such as caffeine, that lead to low blood sugar after an initial 'high'. Certain artificial sweeteners can also have this effect on people who are sensitive to them, by stimulating the secretion of a small amount of insulin. Finally, alcohol can also destabilize your blood sugar levels and cause intense hunger, especially if taken in excess on an empty stomach.

Keeping a food diary will help you to build up a clear picture of your eating habits. Use it to identify any foods that may be causing your problem by relating the times you are hungry or have cravings to what you have eaten that day. You will probably find that a starchy carbohydrate with a high glycaemic index is the main culprit, bread being the most common, but potatoes, white rice, and sugary foods are also among the usual suspects.

Your food diary can also help you find out if any sweeteners or stimulants in beverages or dietary supplements are causing your low blood sugar levels, or whether it is due to strenuous exercise or alcohol consumption.

2 DIETARY CHANGES

If poor choice of foods is the cause of your problem, the first step to take is to cut down on processed foods. Increase your intake of foods that are going to keep you going for longer without feeling hungry, and cut down on those that release energy very quickly and leave you more hungry and out of steam. Broadly speaking, this means eating more whole foods and reducing your intake of those containing processed and refined ingredients, right across all food groups (see page 134) but

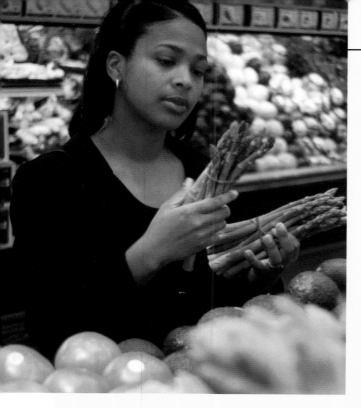

especially carbohydrates. You should also cut down on processed meats and substitute them with fresh or cooked cuts of meat, poultry or fish.

You can also use the glycaemic index to help you substitute your problem foods with those that have a lower GI. Lower-GI foods will result in more stable blood sugar levels so that you feel less hungry, have fewer cravings between meals, remain mentally alert and avoid mood swings. If your diet is very carbohydrate-heavy, you should consider eating more protein. Protein, especially from animal sources, is very filling when combined with carbohydrate, and can reduce the GI of the carbohydrate by slowing down its absorption in your small intestine.

Another good way to make your meals more filling is to eat more vegetables. The denser varieties with a low water content, such as broccoli, cauliflower and leeks, are especially helpful because they are high in bulk and therefore very filling. Try gradually replacing the starchy element of your meals with vegetables – you will feel fuller and at the same time reduce your calorie intake.

3 FOOD PREPARATION

Pay closer attention to the way your food is prepared and cooked before you eat it, because this can affect the speed with which you digest and absorb it. In the case of carbohydrates, anything that alters their fibre structure and content will alter their glycaemic index. Excessive cooking, chopping, puréeing and liquidizing can increase the GI, as does the canning process.

Vegetables should be crunchy and pasta al dente. Cook your own beans and pulses if possible.

CONSISTENCY COUNTS

The consistency of food can determine how filling it will be. Fluids are the least filling, followed by semi-solids, with solid food being the most filling. So sugary drinks are likely to have little value in delaying hunger and do nothing other than add to your daily calorie intake.

4 AVOID STIMULANTS

The most commonly encountered stimulant is the caffeine found in tea, coffee and many soft drinks. Replace these with low-caffeine alternatives such as green or white tea, or use herbal or decaffeinated varieties. Avoid dietary supplements that contain caffeine or other stimulants (such as guarana or taurine) that can affect blood sugar levels, and cut out artificial sweeteners if you think you may be sensitive to them.

5 EXERCISE JUDICIOUSLY

Strenuous aerobic exercise can make you feel very hungry, so to avoid this, either make sure you have a small, light snack just before or after you exercise, or rethink your exercise routine. Taking longer periods of moderate intensity exercise, such as walking, is less likely to stimulate your appetite than short-duration, high-intensity exercise such as running.

6 CUT DOWN ON ALCOHOL

Alcohol can increase hunger and food cravings in two ways, by causing low blood sugar and affecting your brain's appetite centre. Try eating something, ideally carbohydrate, just before or with your drink to delay its absorption and cushion the impact on your bloodstream.

TRIPLE WHAMMY

Fat plays little part in appetite control during weight loss. Although fat slows down your digestion when you eat it as part of a meal, the excess calories it provides will hinder weight loss. What's more fat, when combined with refined carbohydrates in foods such as pastries, cakes and confectionery, actually increases your overall insulin secretion and so promotes body fat storage. Such foods are a triple whammy for weight loss because they are high in calories, lead to greater fat storage and are more likely to increase, not control, your appetite.

PRACTICAL TIPS

Keep well-hydrated. Dehydration can cause lethargy and so occasionally people reach for more food to perk them up, when in fact what they need is more fluid.

• Use vinegar and lemon juice in dressings and sauces because acidity can lower the GI of a food and delay its absorption.

• Avoid ready-made or other foods that require reheating. Foods that can be eaten without reheating retain more of their fibrous structure and bulk and are more filling.

APPETITE AND YOUR SENSES

The feelings of hunger, satiation and satiety, which form the main part of your body's appetite control system, are called 'neurohumeral' mechanisms because they are triggered in your brain by a combination of nerve and hormone signals. These signals are produced by your body in response to your blood sugar levels and the amount and type of food you have eaten.

The neurohumeral system is relatively slow-acting, but the food you eat can affect your appetite in other, more immediate ways, via 'sensorineural' mechanisms, which involve your senses and nerve signals sent to your brain from your eyes, nose and mouth. These mechanisms respond to information about the sight, smell, taste and mouth-feel of the food, and they influence the appetite centre of your brain to either increase or suppress your desire to eat.

Sensorineural signals travel instantaneously, so their effect is immediate and kicks in before your slower neurohumeral mechanisms of satiation and satiety have begun to act. They are also very powerful, and can override the neurohumeral system even when it does become activated, which is why you sometimes want to eat even when you are not hungry and long after you are full.

Visual form and smell alert your eyes and nose, which send signals to the brain and get the appetite going long before you taste anything.

The sensorineural system is there to help us decide quickly if food is fit for

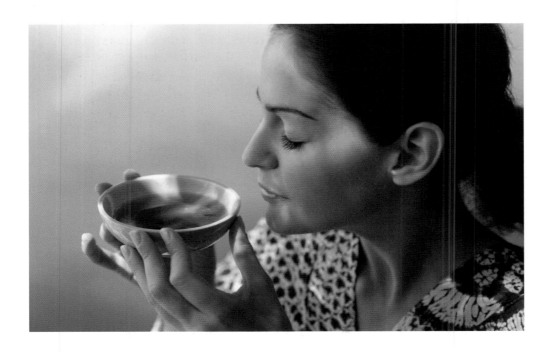

consumption and likely to contain energy, or if it may be harmful or toxic. We are instinctively repelled by the sight and smell of rotten food, while sweet-smelling foods with fresh, vibrant colours are attractive. Our distant ancestors had to forage for food, and those who couldn't tell good food from bad would have died out pretty quickly. Thanks to this evolutionary pressure, our ability to pick out high calorie, non-toxic foods has been so perfected that, even at a distance, the sight or smell of them can stimulate our appetites, while unpleasant-looking or bad-smelling foods are an immediate turnoff.

THE IRRESISTIBLE DESIRE FOR DESSERTS

The delicious taste of food can produce what is called 'post-ingestive hunger'. This is when you find that you crave food, often something sweet, straight after finishing a substantial meal. This was once thought to be due to a surge of insulin lowering blood sugar levels, but it happens too quickly for that and it is actually related to the sensory appeal of food, especially highly palatable food that overstimulates your taste buds.

THE IMPORTANCE OF TASTE

Your senses assess the overall appeal of a food from its taste, texture and mouth-feel, as well as its visual form and aroma, so if any of these properties is enhanced it is likely to increase both the food's desirability and your appetite.

The sensation of taste is particularly important. When you eat food that is palatable, the signals from your taste buds reach areas of your brain that act as reward centres. These create feelings of pleasure, and encourage eating by stimulating your appetite centre and overriding any other signals arriving there, including those that tell it that you've eaten enough. In other words, if food tastes very good, the positive feedback from reward centres can encourage you to keep eating well after you feel full and even when you are not particularly hungry. The effect may be so overwhelmingly powerful that it is unlikely to stop until you have eaten a substantial amount of calories and feel uncomfortably full.

The palatability of food is greatly increased by the presence of fat or sweetness. Fat improves mouth-feel, and sweetness in food is something we are biologically driven to seek out because it signifies a high energy content. Even very young babies can detect sweetness and are instantly deterred by bitterness, a reflex to protect them from eating foods that may be toxic.

Our reward centres have evolved to be mildly activated by the natural sweetness in fruits and vegetables which, being full of natural fibre and slow-release carbohydrates, also fill you up and so have no overall effect on your appetite. Today, though, most of the sugars in the foods we eat are highly purified and concentrated. Their intense sweetness produces rapid stimulation of the reward centres, a stimulation so strong that it easily overrides any feedback signals trying to limit food intake.

MECHANISM OF TASTE

Taste buds are found mainly along the sides of the tongue; the centre does not hold many taste receptors. Taste buds are actually special nerve endings that are able to detect different tastes. The receptors for bitterness lie at the back of the tongue and those for sweetness at the front. Between the two are the receptors for salty and sour. The nerve impulses generated when detecting the tastes are transported to the brain; smell also plays a very important role.

5 Filiform papillae
Are the smallest of the papillae and are scattered over the front two-thirds of the tongue. They are threadlike and are not associated with taste buds.

6 Fungiform papillae
Are the most numerous along the edges and tip of the tongue. They are mushroom-shaped, as their name indicates. Each one has five or so taste buds.

7 Circumvallate papillae
Are the largest of the papillae and are circular in shape. A circumvallate papilla can be associated with up to 1000 taste buds.

1 Bitter
2 Sour
3 Salty
4 Sweet

TONGUE

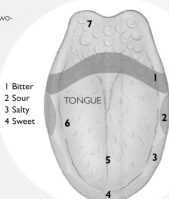

When the taste of sweetness is combined with the mouth-feel of fat, as it is in sugary, high-fat foods, the effect on the reward centres is even greater, creating a forceful incentive to eating that is extremely hard to resist. These high-calorie, low-fibre foods are made with fast-release carbohydrates that are easily chewed and rapidly delivered to your stomach, so they simply bypass the natural satiation and satiety mechanisms that try to limit your food intake. These properties make such foods highly 'addictive' (see pages 128–32), which can lead to grazing, where one sugar hit leaves you craving another a short time later, and to passive overconsumption, where you regularly consume an excessive amount of calories without realizing it.

Grazing also appears to activate, and be perpetuated by, reward centres that respond to the very action of eating. When you start eating, these reward centres tell you to keep going and once

SWEET LOW-CALORIE FATTENERS

Using artificial sweeteners in place of sugar can, paradoxically, cause overeating. These sweeteners may have fewer calories, but they have the same concentrated sweetness as the calorie-rich sugars that turn on your reward centres, so they stimulate your appetite in exactly the same way. In fact, because sweeteners improve taste but have no satiation or satiety value, foods made with them often do not satisfy and you may actually end up eating more.

activated, they remain 'switched on' for about twenty minutes. When the food you're eating is also unnaturally palatable but doesn't make you feel full, the result is an almost overwhelming incentive to continue eating, which is how eating one biscuit tempts you to finish the packet. You have to make a conscious decision to stop, otherwise by the time the packet is empty and/or you feel full, you will most likely have consumed a disproportionately large number of calories. That is why it is so important to control the portion size when you eat high-calorie foods.

Dieting appears to make your reward centres more sensitive to the sensory appeal of food and the oral pleasure of eating. At the same time, the hunger of dieting can lower your 'acceptability threshold' so that foods that you would normally find unpalatable become more acceptable. These effects can continue when you begin to eat normally again, and this may explain why people who

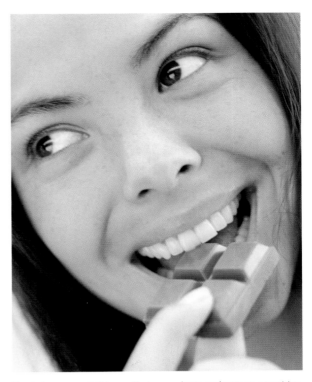

Food that tastes delicious affects your brain and sets up a positive reward feedback loop that encourages you to eat even after you feel full.

have yo-yo dieted find their appetites more and more difficult to control. Indeed, research has shown that overweight people who have lost weight successfully in the past now have a greater preference for sugary, high-fat foods.

It has also been suggested that some people who seem predisposed to gain weight may simply have been born with more sensitive reward centres. Studies have also found that overweight people have a greater preference for high-fat foods than the population as a whole, especially when fat is combined with sweetness or with salt in savoury foods. However, it is uncertain if this preference is genetic or whether it has been acquired, because humans have a great capacity to learn and to develop a taste for different foods. It is possible to acquire a liking for high-fat or sugary foods very quickly, but, with persistence, you can also steer your preferences away from such foods.

APPETITE AND ENVIRONMENT

Of all the forces that influence your eating habits, those arising from your physical and social environment are among the least obvious but most powerful. Your family, friends, job, finances and personal circumstances can all influence your food choices and appetite, as can advertising, retailing, the price of food and current trends and culture. These forces shape your eating behaviour, appetite and dietary choices throughout your lifetime, from the moment you are born, and recognizing and challenging them may help you to break free from negative and counterproductive patterns of eating that have prevented you from losing weight.

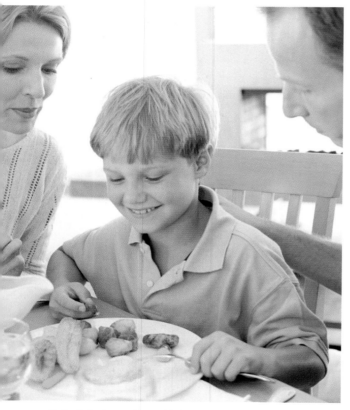

Eating behaviour is learned behaviour that begins in childhood. Not only can our parents determine the foods we will like to eat but also when and how we eat them.

SOCIAL CONDITIONING

We are all born with an intrinsic ability to control our food intake but throughout our childhoods we are told what to eat, when to eat and how much to eat, so we lose touch with our natural hunger and satiety cues. Instead, we rely more and more on external cues, so that as adults we often eat not out of hunger but when it is socially acceptable to do so.

In fact, much of our eating behaviour as adults has its roots in childhood. Children learn to share the same lifestyles and dietary tastes as their immediate carers, both good and bad. If you are a child growing up in a Japanese household, you will develop different choices and eating styles than you would in an Indian, American or French household.

Throughout childhood, we also come to attach symbolism such as sinfulness or purity to certain foods, and give them emotional value if they are used as reward or punishment or as a way of dealing with physical or emotional pain or distress. We may even associate certain foods with important events, because many social occasions, including birthdays, weddings, religious festivals and parties involve food. So eating gains a social significance as an expression of hospitality and a way of bonding, nurturing and cementing relationships. Families that eat together, stay together!

CHANGING LIFESTYLES

As adults, we like to think we have greater freedom in our dietary choices, but in fact these are greatly limited by our personal and family circumstances, our jobs, our finances and even the amount of free time we have. Changes in our lifestyles have, on the whole, placed greater demands on our time and this, together with the rapid expansion in food retailing, means that fewer people now actually cook and eat three meals a day. Most of us now rely more and more on manufactured and ready-made foods, takeaways and restaurant food for a substantial proportion of our daily calorie intake.

This is not surprising, given the ready availability and choice of food outlets and supermarkets, especially in urban areas. With so much competition, however, manufacturers have found increasingly clever and subtle ways of encouraging us not only to spend more on their products, but also to eat more. For them, quite simply, if we eat more, we buy more.

THE HAZARDS OF A WESTERN DIET
Population studies have consistently shown that when people from rural areas in developing nations migrate to Western countries, their rates of obesity and related health problems gradually rise to levels similar to those of their host communities. At the same time, many countries (such as Japan) that have relatively recently adopted a largely Western diet and lifestyle are seeing increasing levels of obesity and related disorders. These particularly affect younger people, who are more vulnerable to the advertising and marketing of Western-style foods and drinks.

THE BUSINESS OF CONSUMPTION

Food retailers, manufacturers and restaurant chains spend millions researching our shopping and eating habits so they can find ways to increase their sales. Their primary motive is, after all, to make money. They make foods that appeal directly to your palate and your pocket, often by using cheap, mass-produced ingredients such as refined carbohydrates (sugar, fat and white flour) and using artificial additives to improve the taste, texture and sensory appeal of the food.

These tactics make their products irresistibly delicious and easily affordable, but also very high in calories and generally not very filling, so you can and do eat more. Remember, whether it's snack foods, haute cuisine or fast foods, it is not really profitable to make foods that are filling or that keep you sated. To the food industry, it makes better commercial sense if you eat all the biscuits rather than just two, or order three courses at the restaurant instead of one. And when there is little or no nutritional information about a product, or when its sugar or fat content is disguised by complex terminology and misleading labelling, can you really help making poor dietary choices?

The atmosphere in which food is sold is also gently manipulated to arouse your appetite – think of the aroma of freshly brewed coffee in restaurants, or of freshly baked bread or doughnuts in supermarkets, or the ways in which stores arrange their goods to encourage impulse-buying. Some restaurants and bars subtly alter their background music as the evening wears on, because when the music becomes faster, you eat and drink faster. Careful lighting can enhance the colours of foods in stores or create conducive atmospheres in restaurants – people tend to eat more in an intimate, softly lit environment than in a bright, open room where they feel more vulnerable to gazing eyes. Some restaurants even display images of meals carefully prepared by food stylists to stimulate your appetite.

Retailers also target your intrinsic sense of value by discounting prices and promoting special offers, such as '3 for the price of 2', 'buy one, get one free', or extra points on loyalty cards, while restaurants offer cut-price 'meal deals' such as set menus at discounted prices or bigger portion sizes. These gimmicks have the sole intention of encouraging you to buy more, and when you buy more you tend to consume more. Three packets of biscuits rarely last three times as long as one, and one portion size does not fit all.

ADVERTISING AND MARKETING

The most powerful weapon that food manufacturers and retailers have in their arsenal is advertising. It aims not only to appeal to our senses and tastes but also to change our beliefs, attitudes, desires and aspirations. It is particularly effective when it targets children and teenagers. Advertising and 'branding' can elevate products to cult status, encouraging you to eat foods you would not normally consume.

Food and drinks companies pay for approximately 80 percent of total advertising, and three-quarters of that is for foods high in fat and/or sugar. This is grossly out of proportion to recommended consumption levels, and unfortunately not counterbalanced by advertising for healthy foods such as fruit and vegetables. The retail food industry would claim that it is simply providing products that reflect consumer demand. However, the odds are greatly stacked in their favour. By their very presence, these foods foster complacency, as they become an increasingly attractive alternative to buying, preparing and cooking your own food. These intense advertising and marketing campaigns give added legitimacy to such choices, making them socially acceptable lifestyle options.

Although in any given individual several factors together result in weight gain, there is little doubt that the increased availability and accessibility of palatable high-energy foods, backed by an extremely powerful retail food industry, has helped to create an obesity-creating environment in which overconsumption has become virtually inescapable.

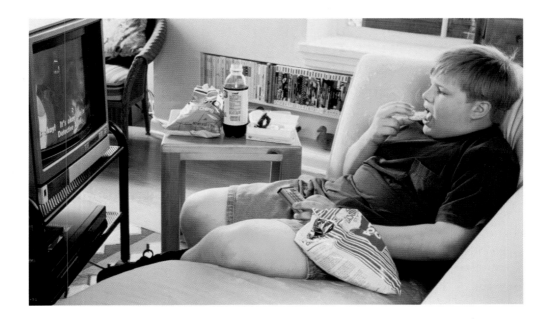

Children are unwitting victims of food and drink advertising that creates an 'obesogenic' environment in which overconsumption is the norm.

NATIONAL TRADITIONS

The foods we choose to eat can also reflect your nationality, locality, religious upbringing, cultural heritage, social conscience, and the social class from which you originate or to which you aspire – in essence, they form an important part of your identity. Fish and chips and roast beef and Yorkshire pudding are part of what defines being British, just as sushi and sashimi define the Japanese and pasta and pizza, the Italians. The cooking style, the times of meals, the order in which foods are eaten and their taste, texture and consistency all vary from nation to nation, as do the types of food and food combinations that are widely available. Changing the relatively unhealthy diet of the average Scot to the more healthy eating habits of the average Japanese would imply changing people and a large part of their cultural identity and heritage. Remember that these factors may limit the extent to which you are willing to make dietary changes yourself.

CLIMATE

Climate also plays a part in national cultures and eating habits, and changing weather can affect your appetite and which foods you prefer at different times of the year. Hot and hearty stews and mashed potatoes lose their appeal on a hot summer day, just as cold salads and fruits are unappetizing in the bleak midwinter. Climate can also affect your mood, energy and activity levels. Cold weather and reduced daylight hours, for example, can increase your desire for sugary, high-fat comfort foods, so trying to lose weight at such times may naturally prove more difficult.

DISORDERED EATING

An erratic pattern of food intake, disordered eating is what happens when the amount of food a person eats, and the times at which he or she eat it, vary greatly from one day to another. Generally, the pattern is unpredictable, but usually involves eating large amounts of food in short periods of time, interspersed with long periods of eating very little.

JACKIE was working as a kindergarten teacher when she attended the clinic, having tried unsuccessfully to lose weight. She could manage to eat sensibly throughout the day but less so towards the evening, at which time she would find herself overeating and occasionally bingeing. Looking at her food diary, the pattern that emerged was one of feast and famine. She left home early to commute to work, so she would often skip breakfast and then have a light lunch such as a salad, or often just a yogurt, or a piece of fruit. By afternoon and early evening, she would generally be quite hungry, so she occasionally bought sweets or crisps to eat on the way home. Once home, she would find it hard to control her appetite, eating anything that was immediately to hand, followed by dinner and an array of often fatty or sugary snacks, right up until bedtime. She complained of feeling tired during the day, and so she felt that taking additional exercise was out of the question. She also had difficulty sleeping at night.

WHAT CAUSES IT?

Patterns of eating like Jackie's (see left) are very common, particularly the tendency to skip breakfast. Working unsocial shift patterns, having to get to work very early in the morning, or preparing the children for school, often mean that it is easier to wait until later to eat. Skipping lunch and 'saving up' most of the day's calorie intake for the evening is also quite common. It may occur, for example, because of a lack of time at work or because healthy foods are unavailable during the day, and sometimes it may simply be due to the expense of eating away from home.

For some people, however, there are psychological reasons for eating in this way. Busy jobs and lifestyles distract them from thinking about food and eating, so they find that they can control their appetites very easily when they have plenty of other things to do. And sometimes they don't trust themselves to be able to eat less in the evening, so they compensate for this by depriving themselves of food during the day. They may even consider extra snacks later as a reward: 'I didn't have lunch, so I can afford to indulge!' Then they feel guilty about overeating, and so try to make amends by eating less the next day, and so it goes on. Whatever the initial reasons, many people soon become caught up in this cycle of feast and fasting.

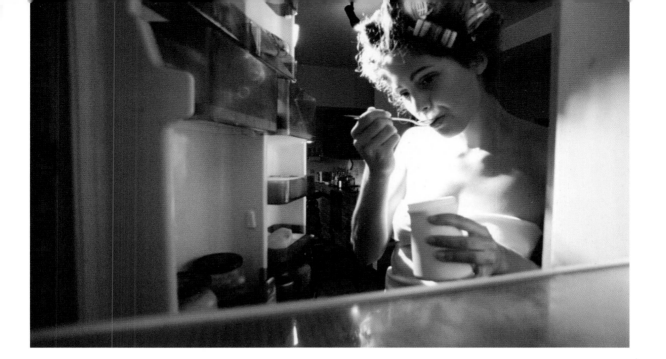

THE CONSEQUENCES

Unfortunately, this pattern of eating lots of food in between long periods of eating little or nothing can trigger an internal defence mechanism that is actually designed to stop you from losing weight. It can even make you gain weight in the long term.

Eating very little during the day, for instance by going without breakfast and then having a simple snack lunch at work, can actually make you gain weight. It does this by slowing down your metabolism and by making you more likely to overeat when you get home.

This defence mechanism has developed over the millennia of human evolution, and its purpose is to increase your chances of survival during periods of famine, which in the past were by far the greatest threat to our ancestors. It enables your body to function without using up too many valuable calories when food is scarce, and in the process it makes you more efficient at storing fat when food is readily available. This is to make you better prepared to survive any future famines. Your body is designed to store fat and to use it only when absolutely necessary, and so the more it senses potential danger, in the form of a lack of food, the more it tries and the better it gets at stubbornly hanging on to your fat reserves. The increase in your mental drive to obtain food at this time is also part of this survival instinct. Hunger and cravings are natural biological urges that make you want to eat. They are there to regulate your eating and are very difficult to resist. In fact, trying to resist them only makes them stronger, so that ultimately you may end up eating more than normal.

When you don't eat properly for a long time, your blood sugar drops and so your brain generates hunger cues and cravings in an attempt to prompt you to eat, before your body taps into your fat or protein reserves. If you still don't eat, your body then

EATING DISORDERS

Anorexia nervosa and bulimia are the result of complex and poorly understood causes, however, once a sufferer starts to link body image and eating with mood and self-esteem, he or she embarks on a path that normally requires professional care.

Stress, depression, low self-esteem. A morbid obsession with fatness.

Severe dieting. Overactivity. Obsession with exercise.

Severe weight loss. Fatigue, weakness. Poor skin and hair. Continued obsession with weight.

Uncontrolled binge eating followed by induced vomiting.

Severe psychological disorders – professional advice is needed.

enters a semi-starvation mode during which your metabolism slows down in order to save calories. This can make you feel physically tired and cold. You may find it difficult to concentrate, and you may lack motivation or feel drowsy, moody, and irritable. Your mental focus also shifts towards food, so you may begin to obsess about food and eating in general. Your desire to eat builds up, until eventually you give in to cravings or overeat when food finally becomes available.

At this point, your excessive food intake, combined with the increased 'fuel efficiency' of your body, means that more of this food is going to be stored as body fat. This is especially likely to happen if you overeat in the evening, when you are also less physically active. Skipping meals, eating irregularly, and overriding your body's hunger cues can create a combination of physical and psychological factors that conspire to prevent you losing weight.

DISORDERED EATING IN QUESTION

Looking back at our case history, we can see how Jackie's behaviour prevented her from losing weight. During the day, she used work and other activities to distract her mind so that she could override the natural hunger cues that were prompting her to eat. Her metabolism then slowed right down, so she was probably burning fewer calories even though she was active. She kept herself going for as long as she could with sheer willpower, despite feeling tired and lacking energy.

By the end of the day, her appetite had really built up and, as she also had less to occupy her, she found it much harder to control her food intake. Eventually, she would give in to cravings for high-calorie snacks such as chocolates and biscuits, and then generally overeat. Her night-time eating more than made up for the lack of food during the day, and so her overall daily calorie intake was actually quite high. And as she took in most of her food over a fairly small period of time, during which she was also much less active than she had been earlier in the day, much of it was converted to body fat. She had triggered her body's natural defences into trying to stop her from losing weight. By bedtime, she felt bloated and somewhat guilty about her overeating.

At the same time, because her body was trying to digest all the food she had eaten, her metabolism picked up and so she also found it harder to sleep.

Regularly eating in this way can, over time, condition your body to become better at storing and holding onto body fat, and it prompts your appetite to become more and more intense. This makes weight loss even harder to achieve, both physiologically and psychologically. The solution to this problem is to follow a recovery programme that changes your eating habits and returns your metabolism to normal.

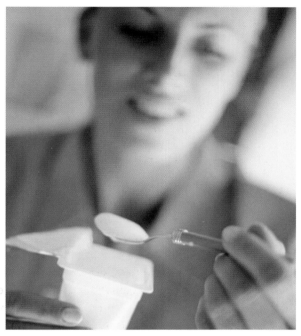

Prevent your metabolism from slowing down during the day by eating something at least every three or four hours, but avoid foods that are high in sugar or fat.

SOLVING THE PROBLEM

The main aim of the recovery programme (see pages 82–3) is to learn to spread your calorie intake more evenly over the course of the whole day. Eventually, this may mean eating three main meals a day with small snacks in between, or perhaps eating five smaller meals. At the beginning, however, simply establishing a more regular and reliable pattern of eating is much more important than attempting to restrict your calorie intake. Continue eating the same foods, but spread your intake over the whole day – you will not achieve long-term weight loss until you learn to eat in a regular and predictable manner.

HUNGER AND SATIETY

Try to become more aware of hunger cues and regulate your eating accordingly. Use the index on page 83 as a guide, and eat when you are beginning to feel hungry (stage 3 on the Hunger Index) and stop when you reach stage 3 on the Satiety Index – comfortable but satisfied. Don't make the mistake of waiting until you are very hungry before starting to eat, because you are then much more likely to overeat or to give in to cravings for sweets and biscuits.

Disordered Eating Recovery Programme

1 FIND THE CAUSE

Before you try to make any changes to your eating behaviour, you must try to understand why you are eating in this way. Is it for practical reasons of time and food availability, or are there psychological reasons? It is important to understand your behaviour because you need to identify the cause of your problem before you can begin to solve it. Practical reasons have practical solutions, whereas psychological ones require relearning of behaviour, which may take more time and effort.

2 UNDERSTAND THE PHYSIOLOGY

Eating at regular times will enable your body to associate hunger with meal times, and when it learns that feelings of hunger will soon be followed by a meal, it won't be prompted to trigger its fat-storing defence mechanism. Connecting hunger to meal times will also allow you, in time, to regulate meal and portion size to the predicted time of your next meal.

Do not skip breakfast, it is an important meal that kick-starts your metabolism in the morning, and don't skip lunch because doing so can lead to overeating at night. Try not to go for longer than three to four hours during the day without eating something, even a light snack such as an apple or a small pot of yogurt. This will prevent your metabolism from slowing down when you are active, and prevent your appetite from building up too much, which can lead to overeating later in the day or at night.

> **FAT FACT**
>
> **STARVING YOURSELF LEADS TO MUSCLE LOSS**
>
> Did you know that when you do not eat for a long time, you tend to lose muscle as well as fat? Muscle burns about 40 calories per hour per kilogram at rest, whereas fat burns only about 5 calories. So it is more 'costly' for the body to maintain muscle tissue than fat, and in starvation mode it tends to shed the expensive muscle as well as the fat. Losing muscle slows your metabolism permanently and so you burn fewer calories throughout the day. It also makes you more prone to gain weight in the future, and this is what happens when people try to lose weight too quickly.

3 SET GOALS

Begin to institute small changes in your behaviour. If you normally don't eat breakfast, start doing so by eating something very light every morning – a piece of toast, a bowl of cereal or a piece of fruit. Approach lunch in a similar manner. Make small changes that you can build on, don't expect to make too many changes all at once, and, in the early days don't worry too much about your weight.

4 MAKE DIETARY CHANGES

Once you have become used to eating at regular times, you will find it easier to make the dietary changes (see pages 67–8) that will help you to lose weight. When meal times are predictable and you become better at relying on your body's feelings of hunger and satiety to tell you when and how much to eat (see box, below), eating the right foods will almost automatically lead to weight loss. You will feel fuller for longer and so be able to eat less, but you will still find you have more energy during the day, for work, exercise and other activities. Your mood and concentration will improve, and you also will find that you sleep more comfortably at night.

5 LIKELY PROBLEMS

Many people who have been eating in an erratic way for a long time find eating more regular meals scary: 'What if I eat breakfast and lunch and still can't control my eating at night as well? I'm going to put on even more weight!' Unless you are overeating for emotional reasons, this won't happen. Your natural mechanisms for regulating food intake – hunger and satiety – are actually very good at their job. But problems can arise if you lose touch with this internal mechanism and start to rely on your own conscious will or external cues to tell you what, when, and how much to eat. These are much less reliable methods of regulating food intake.

PRACTICAL TIPS

• **Take a packed lunch prepared at home to work – this can save you money as well as ensuring that you get a healthy meal in the middle of the day. Don't forget your own healthy snacks, salad dressings and drinks.**
• **If you have a long journey home, have a small healthy snack before leaving work – you will then be less likely to overeat when you get home.**
• **Do not go shopping when hungry at the end of the day. You are much more likely to buy unhealthy, calorie-rich snacks and meals.**
• **Go prepared with a shopping list so that you can quickly pick up what you need and avoid browsing, which often leads to impulse buying.**

HUNGER INDEX	SATIETY INDEX
1 Very hungry	1 Empty
2 Hungry	2 Not satisfied
3 Starting to feel hungry	3 Comfortable but satisfied
4 Peckish	4 Full
5 Not hungry	5 Uncomfortably full

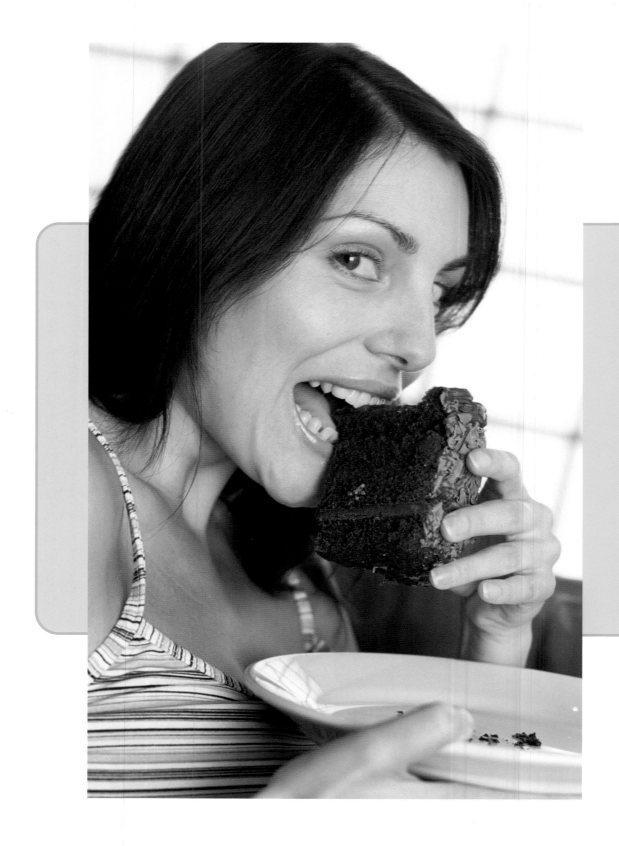

3

CAUSES OF OVEREATING

PSYCHOLOGICAL ISSUES

The mechanisms that control our appetites, such as our blood sugar levels and the sight, smell and taste of our food, are overlaid by many complex psychological influences. These include our memories, thoughts, emotions and moods, and they can affect our eating behaviour in many unexpected ways.

THE FLAWED PSYCHOLOGY OF DIETING

The growth of the dieting culture in society has led to the emergence of an interesting paradox: dieting as a cause of obesity. Apart from producing metabolic changes in the body, which may contribute to future weight gain, the act of dieting — losing weight by consciously depriving yourself of food — can in some people trigger psychological changes and disordered eating behaviour that may, in the long term, result in weight gain.

Research is littered with reports of abnormal eating behaviour in men, women and children after periods of semi-starvation, for example, among people who have been marooned on expeditions, the survivors of prisoner-of-war camps, and people who have lived through famines or wartime food shortages. Even when food became plentiful again, many remained obsessed with it, had rapid and voracious eating patterns, and felt a lack of control over and distress about the amounts they ate. They complained of feeling hungry even after large meals, and admitted to scavenging, hiding and hoarding food and binge eating. They also reported cravings for sweet, sugary and fatty foods, which they ate in isolation and secrecy.

The effect that food deprivation can have on behaviour was nicely demonstrated by a study, carried out in Minnesota in the 1940s, in which a group of men were placed on a moderately low-calorie diet of 1500 calories per day. This is still a fairly decent energy intake, and yet in just ten weeks the researchers observed major personality changes in the men and in their behaviour as their weight loss progressed. The men became increasingly obsessed with food in their thoughts, conversations and choice of reading material. They began smuggling and hoarding food, which they ate in secrecy, and even appeared to gain satisfaction from watching others eat.

The men also showed changes in mood, expressing more anger, hostility

> **FAT FALLACY**
>
> **EMOTIONAL PROBLEMS CAUSE OBESITY**
>
> Emotional problems such as low self-esteem, anxiety and depression are more likely to be a result of obesity than a cause of it, because most of them improve with weight loss. On the whole, overweight people have no more psychological disorders than the general population, and there is no evidence of a particular personality type associated with an increased risk of obesity.

and pessimism, and they developed greater levels of anxiety and depression, which continued well over six months after the trial had ended. At that time, they also confessed to episodes of uncontrollable binge eating, distress with overeating, and cravings for sugary and fatty foods. Several actually succumbed to the urge to vomit or purge after episodes of uncontrolled eating while some, on regaining their lost weight, reported feeling unhappy about their physique, in particular their abdomen and buttocks, despite having no previous history of anxiety over body shape.

Does this seem vaguely familiar? This and other studies confirm what many people who have dieted before already know, which is that dieting makes you moody, irritable and preoccupied with food. And once you end your diet, you binge on all the foods you had banned. Then you not only gain even more weight than you had lost, but also develop patterns of negative thinking involving guilt, shame and depression about eating and your body size. These changes are all part of your body's natural and instinctive survival mechanism, and when you diet by drastically cutting down your calorie intake, you trigger this reaction.

THE HAZARDS OF STARVATION DIETS

If you suddenly eat less than normal and go hungry to lose weight, particularly if you skip meals, your body thinks you are experiencing a famine. It then reacts physically by slowing down your metabolism to preserve precious calories, and psychologically by increasing your preoccupation with food in an attempt to intensify your biological drive to obtain and eat it. Psychological recovery after such a stressful event can take a long time, so when you finally end your diet, your mental focus remains on food. This is to make sure you replenish your lost fat reserves so that your body is better prepared should you encounter famine again. When you actively try to reduce your fat reserves, your body reacts by trying to increase them even more.

A large and prolonged drop in your average daily calorie intake creates a constant internal battle, fought between the conscious part of your brain that wants you to eat less and the instinctive part that wills you to eat more. This battle can lead to cycles of bingeing, guilt and shame followed by a strengthened resolve to diet even harder, and so every time you go on a 'starvation' diet to lose weight, these psychological drives intensify. Then you can easily get into a cycle of yo-yo dieting in which your thoughts and behaviour become increasingly dominated by food and eating.

These thought and behaviour patterns, together with the physiological changes in your body, lead paradoxically to weight gain in the long term. The psychological changes that occur may also play a role in the development or the perpetuation of a number of eating disorders, including binge eating disorder (BED), compulsive eating or perhaps even anorexia and bulimia. Trying to lose weight quickly by severely restricting your food intake and consciously overriding your body's hunger cues is counterproductive and must be avoided.

RESTRAINED EATING

A more moderate form of dieting behaviour, called restrained eating, is seen in people who are perpetually on a diet. Restrained eaters may have yo-yo dieted in the past, or they may be genetically predisposed to weight gain. They are usually around normal weight, but they have to remain vigilant and consciously restrain themselves from overeating on a daily, meal-to-meal, basis to keep their weight at a desirable level.

Restrained eaters are constantly fighting psychologically against their biological drives to eat, and as a result they develop abnormal eating behaviours to control their food intake and become preoccupied with food and eating. They also have a tendency to 'disinhibited' eating. When restrained eaters are forced or triggered by outside events to temporarily come off their diets, they don't just eat a little bit more. Their eating becomes disinhibited as they totally abandon all moderation and overeat, while reassuring themselves that it's OK because they will soon restart their diets.

The idea that the diet will return in the near future appears to reinforce the motivation to act against their self-imposed restraint, a process called 'counter-regulation'. The stricter the diet, the greater the loss of control, and temporarily suspending restraint releases the underlying desire to eat. If you have dieted in the past you can probably relate to this pattern of thinking and behaviour, in which a small lapse in dietary control can quickly turn into an all-out but short-lived binge. Trigger factors include tasting small amounts of highly palatable foods that have been restricted, the sight or smell of well-liked foods, other people overeating, the anticipation of forthcoming high-food-intake occasions and emotional distress.

Dietary restraint can, therefore, increase your desire and responsiveness to specific foods and make you more sensitive to your emotions or to environmental stimuli. These can trigger a loss of dietary control and cause overeating. This is how dieting can lead to weight gain in the long term. Such a chronic battle to restrain your appetite and eating against powerful biological drives is always difficult to sustain, and can be lost if your will breaks down or weakens under pressure, especially if it is for prolonged periods of time during traumatic life events or emotionally disturbing circumstances.

DISAPPOINTING RESULTS

Diets that rely on deliberate self-restraint to produce weight loss have poor long-term results. Many people fail to lose any weight with this approach and of those who do, 95 percent regain the weight within a year. Other data shows that there are links between increasing levels of obesity, a rising incidence of bingeing, and increasing levels of dieting. There is also a greater prevalence of obesity among women who use self-restraint when they try to lose weight.

THE HEALTH RISKS LINKED TO ANOREXIA NERVOSA

1 Hair
Gets thinner as a result of hormone changes and a lack of nutrients. At the same time, a fine downy hair (lanugo) may grow on the body.

2 Teeth
Are gradually worn away by repeated self-induced vomiting, which causes decay, tooth loss and degeneration of the jawbone.

3 Heart
Tissue is damaged by the low intake of protein, vitamins and minerals, leading to disorders.

4 Breasts
Revert to pre-pubescent size because of muscle wasting, loss of body fat and hormone changes.

5 Kidney
Damage and the risk of failure result from long-term malnutrition.

6 Muscles
Are broken down to provide vital energy in order to compensate for the low calorie intake, leading to muscle wasting.

7 Intestines
Suffer long-term disruption to their digestive functions because of a lack of vital nutrients.

8 Skin
Gets very dry and nails become fragile because of disrupted hormone levels and poor diet.

9 Ovaries
Are affected by hormone imbalances leading to cessation of periods (amenorrhoea) and fertility.

10 Bones
Become brittle and fracture easily (osteoporosis) as a result of reduced calcium intake and hormone imbalances.

DYSFUNCTIONAL EATING

Failing to lose weight is always a disappointment, and for some vulnerable people it can be one that's hard to take. For these people, a diet that hasn't worked brings negative feelings ranging from guilt, shame and despair to an increased susceptibility to dysfunctional eating habits such as emotional eating, compulsive overeating and binge eating disorder. It seems that the commonly held view that dieting doesn't work may, in fact, have some legitimacy after all.

COMPULSIVE OVEREATING

Emotional eating, or comfort eating, as it is more commonly known, is eating food not out of physical hunger but as a response to uncomfortable feelings and emotions. In more extreme cases, emotional eating may be associated with a real sense of loss of control over eating, usually referred to as compulsive overeating.

Many people who exhibit such behaviour have difficulty identifying, tolerating, expressing and regulating their feelings. A number of studies have found an increased rate of anxiety and depression among compulsive overeaters, but it remains uncertain if this is the cause or the result. One theory is that eating sweet, sugary carbohydrates improves levels of serotonin in the brain. Serotonin is a chemical that is important in regulating mood and reducing symptoms of anxiety and depression, so overeating may be biologically driven in compulsive overeaters. At present, however, the research remains inconclusive.

Emotional or compulsive overeating is best dealt with by tackling the underlying psychological issues that trigger it, rather than attempting weight loss. This is because when you resolve these issues, regulating your weight often comes more naturally as you learn to recognize the triggers for your overeating and develop alternative coping skills. You can usually help yourself to overcome the problem of emotional eating (see pages 94–9), but if that doesn't work you should seek professional help in the form of psychological counselling and behavioural therapy.

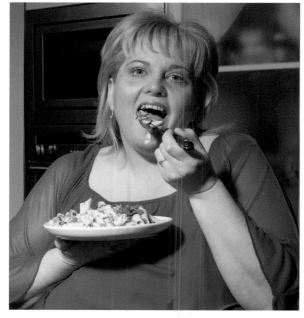

Overeating can be caused by a number of factors including emotional distress. Unless the source of the distress is dealt with, the overeating will continue.

BINGE EATING DISORDER SYMPTOMS

Binge eating disorder is clinically defined by the appearance of two or more of the following symptoms during a 6-month period:

Episodes of eating much more food in a 2-hour period than most people would eat in the same time under similar circumstances.

A sense of loss of control during the episodes.

The episodes are associated with: eating rapidly • eating until uncomfortably full • eating large amounts when not hungry • eating alone because of embarrassment • feeling disgusted, depressed or guilty afterwards • eating late at night • avoiding social situations around food perhaps for fear of loss of control.

Episodes occur at least twice a week.

The episodes are not associated with use of purgatives or laxatives.

BINGE EATING DISORDER (BED)

BED is another condition made worse by dieting. It is a syndrome that affects approximately ten percent of the obese population, and about 40 percent of sufferers are men. Individuals with BED are often overweight or have large or frequent weight fluctuations. They are usually unsuccessful at losing weight or keeping it off, which only serves to intensify their feelings of despair, self-loathing and depression.

Dieting is pointless and only aggravates this condition; the vast majority of sufferers actually develop this disorder after dieting. The best treatment is to seek psychological therapy of some kind, such as cognitive behaviour therapy, psychotherapy, group support or a combination of these. As part of the treatment, individuals are helped to come to terms with their current weight and to gain control over their eating behaviour before attempting weight loss. Addressing problems with body image, and treating anxiety or depression, are also important parts of the recovery programme.

Sufferers of BED often have low self-esteem and are ashamed of their inability to control their behaviour or reason through it. They feel isolated, often thinking that they alone have this disordered pattern of eating. This is definitely not the case; there are many in the same position and plenty of help and support is available.

STRESS AND WEIGHT

The relationship between stress and weight is not as straightforward as it may seem. Although stress has been associated with weight gain, it has also been associated with

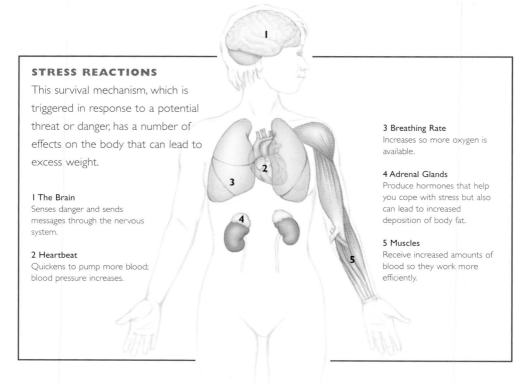

STRESS REACTIONS

This survival mechanism, which is triggered in response to a potential threat or danger, has a number of effects on the body that can lead to excess weight.

1 The Brain
Senses danger and sends messages through the nervous system.

2 Heartbeat
Quickens to pump more blood; blood pressure increases.

3 Breathing Rate
Increases so more oxygen is available.

4 Adrenal Glands
Produce hormones that help you cope with stress but also can lead to increased deposition of body fat.

5 Muscles
Receive increased amounts of blood so they work more efficiently.

weight loss and there is little to suggest that there is a direct cause-and-effect relationship. The body physically reacts to stressful situations instantly by either freezing out of fear, preparing to fight or fleeing as fast as possible. All three reactions release stress hormones including adrenaline and cortisol. Adrenaline raises your heart rate, blood pressure and breathing rate, while increased levels of cortisol have been associated with increased deposition of body fat around the abdomen. The latter has implications for weight and general health, as it is associated with high blood pressure, diabetes, high blood cholesterol and heart disease, and Metabolic Syndrome.

Stress may also contribute to weight gain by acting as an external cue to overeating, especially emotional eating in response to feelings generated by it, such as anger, frustration, anxiety and depression. In individuals showing restrained eating (see pages 88–9), stress can act as a powerful disinhibitor leading to overeating and even bingeing. Similarly, those with BED report increased bingeing in response to stress.

Finally, stress may be an indirect factor in weight gain by eroding your ability to manage your time better. When you are under stress, you often function less effectively both physically and mentally. This can encourage poor eating habits, irregular meal times and increasing reliance on convenience foods and snacks, and leave you with less time to take part in physical activity.

Bear in mind that many of these dysfunctional eating behaviours are widespread and are not restricted to people who have been trying to lose weight. They also occur among people of healthy weight, who can experience episodes of dysfunctional or unhealthy eating as a result of stress.

SYMBOLISM AND BODY SIZE

Body size has come to symbolize certain qualities, both positive and negative. These qualities vary from one society or culture to another, and can directly cause or perpetuate increased weight in some individuals.

We tend to think that Western society, on the whole, stigmatizes overweight individuals with unfavourable character traits such as laziness and greed, but our view of them actually includes a number of qualities that can be quite positive. For example, some men find that being overweight gives them a certain gravitas or presence, which enhances their personal stature. Large men may be associated with strength, machismo, power and dominance, and the term 'heavyweight' is often used to describe men in relation to their jobs, always implying that they are to be taken seriously. In women, too, being overweight is not always a negative because it is associated with nurturing and motherly qualities that can be comforting to some spouses and children. Such positive cultural images can sometimes make people, especially men, reluctant to part with excess weight.

Many cultures also associate being overweight with kindness and gentleness — think of images of Father Christmas, Aunt Jemima or even Colonel Sanders. At the same time, most cultures associate losing weight with ill-health, stress and distress. In those developing countries where being overweight is still representative of wealth, weight loss can suggest financial hardship.

The relationship between size and sexuality is also a complex one. Throughout history, overweight women have symbolized fertility but today, especially in the West, being overweight is more often identified with reduced sexuality. As a result, losing weight increases a woman's sexuality and sexual desirability. However, close family members can become uncomfortable when a woman begins to lose weight and become more attractive. They fear that her increased attractiveness might bring her attention from outsiders, who will compete with them for her affections, so sometimes they try to discourage her from losing weight.

At the same time, some women (and men) may themselves subconsciously use weight to create a psychological and physical barrier between themselves and the outside world, for instance to deflect attention, especially of a sexual nature, from the opposite sex. This may be a reaction to previous traumatic and painful close or sexual relationships, or even to previous sexual abuse or rape, making the individual uncomfortable with their own sexuality or that of others. Regardless of the cause, seeking psychotherapeutic counselling is the only way to approach this issue. Facing and dealing with underlying pain and trauma can help to resolve the subconscious resistance to weight loss that may be the cause of failed attempts in the past.

EMOTIONAL EATING

Most of us have occasionally treated ourselves to a favourite comfort food, such as chocolate or ice cream, to cheer us up when we are feeling low. This is a perfectly normal reaction to a minor setback or disappointment, but for some people it can become a problem. They start using food as a way of coping with difficult feelings, and this emotional eating (also known as comfort eating) becomes a chronic habit that can lead to weight gain or hinder attempts to lose weight.

WHAT CAUSES IT?

Many people instinctively understand emotional eating but often do not realize that they are doing it themselves. We all recognize physical hunger, the inbuilt alarm that tells us we need to eat, but emotional or psychological hunger can be harder to detect and often arises out of an emotional reaction, such as anxiety, anger or sadness, to external triggers or events.

These triggers can be minor day-to-day irritations (such as commuting) that produce chronic stress, or sudden and traumatic life events such as divorce or bereavement. They may also relate to conflicts in present relationships or be due to unresolved issues that stem from past relationships or from childhood. The triggers may be different for each individual but they all arouse uncomfortable emotions, and emotional eating occurs not out of true hunger but as a way of coping with or dulling these emotions.

The act of eating, especially highly palatable, high-fat sweet or savoury foods, appears to act on the reward circuits in the brain that release endorphins, our natural feel-good chemicals. These endorphins 'anaesthetize' the pain and emotional discomfort triggered by unpleasant events or memories.

The pleasant and soothing sensations that eating food generates can simply become another way of comforting ourselves, in the same way that some people use shopping, alcohol, recreational drugs and cigarettes. Indeed, many people gain weight after they give up smoking because they are simply exchanging one coping mechanism for another. People tend to use the tools that are available or that they have learned to use, whether as adults or during childhood, to help block awareness of their pain and distance themselves from their feelings. Sometimes, parents unknowingly condition this behaviour in their children by using food to comfort them, rather than encouraging them to express or talk through their emotions.

Emotional eating tends to occur more commonly at night because there are fewer mental and physical distractions at this time. When people find themselves alone and bored, they are more likely to be mulling over the day's events or thinking ahead to the next day's activities. This is when their worries, fears and frustrations begin to surface, and so they turn to food for comfort.

THE CONSEQUENCES

The consequences of emotional eating depend largely on the extent to which you are using food as a coping mechanism, because it also occurs in people of healthy weight. It can, however, be a genuine cause of weight gain or it may prevent you from losing weight, especially if you are repeatedly consuming high-calorie foods at night when you are also less active.

If you've gained weight because of emotional eating, then trying to lose it by dieting alone, without tackling the underlying feelings and their triggers, can prove extremely difficult and many people repeatedly fail to do so. Unfortunately, gaining weight or failing to achieve a desirable weight can both exacerbate feelings of shame, guilt and disappointment that then stimulate more emotional eating (and sometimes drinking). A vicious cycle can arise in which emotional eating leads to weight gain, followed by vigorous attempts at dieting that ultimately fail. These failures create more negative feelings, prompting more emotional eating as a response and then even greater weight gain.

Anne (see opposite page) showed the classic signs of someone using food as a coping mechanism and was in danger of getting caught up in the vicious cycle of emotional eating, weight gain and failed diets. Her self-confidence had been shattered by her divorce and she was struggling to juggle the responsibilities of children, a job and keeping home. She was encountering stress in many aspects of her daily life while still trying to come to terms with a major life event, and was finding her only comfort late at night, in food. Her failure to control her eating was not only preventing her from losing weight, it was slowly eroding her self-esteem and sense of control over her life, pushing her further towards comfort eating and even more weight gain.

If allowed to spiral out of control, her emotional eating could have led to a destructive pattern of yo-yo dieting that, in turn, may have led eventually to intractable obesity or perhaps to more extreme eating behaviours such as binge eating disorder, compulsive overeating or even bulimia.

Emotional Eating Recovery Programme

I FIND THE CAUSE

The first step on the road to recovery from emotional eating is to find the triggers that set it off for you. There may be several that add up throughout the day or one single trigger, such as an insensitive comment, that give rise to uncomfortable feelings. The triggers may all come from the same source, such as conflict with a partner, or arise from different areas of your life and vary from one day to the next.

Sometimes triggers can be blindingly obvious, but others, like childhood abuse or neglect, or the loss of a loved one long ago, may be hidden under many layers of emotional camouflage. When you overreact to something today, the real cause may in fact be rooted in your past. If you worry when you are away from your partner, perhaps it is because a previous partner betrayed you or because your father had affairs when you were a child. You may therefore need to reflect long and hard on various aspects of your life and ask yourself some searching questions, some of which may unearth many painful truths. Do you have any long-standing and unresolved issues in your present personal or professional life? Are there any memories from your past or events rooted in your childhood that are painful to you and that you prefer not to think about? These may be memories you are trying to bury with food.

Triggers to emotional eating may also arise from purely practical issues that, as in Anne's case, create stress if you are trying to deal with too many responsibilities at once. Perhaps you are caring for someone who is elderly, disabled or has a long-term illness. Or maybe you are frustrated in your job. Is your workload beyond or below your capabilities? Are you unhappy with your choice of career?

You may have to search a little to find the root cause of your emotional eating, and you should remember that triggers are subjective and everyone has his or her own. An event that may seem trivial to one person – being late for an appointment, getting caught in traffic or missing a deadline at work – may cause a lot of anxiety or frustration in another.

As well as identifying your triggers, you have to become aware of what it is you are feeling when you overeat. Many people, after a lifetime of using food to distance themselves from their emotions, have lost touch with them and are

TIME TO SSTOPP

Practice the SSTOPP routine whenever you find yourself about to eat when you're not physically hungry:

- Stop what you are doing;
- Step back in your mind;
- Think about what you are feeling;
- Observe what you are doing;
- Put down the food for a moment and take a deep breath;
- Plan what you can do instead.

This plan of action may give you just enough time to stop yourself from eating unwisely.

COMFORT FOODS

Foods that require some degree of crunching and gnashing, such as pretzels and crisps, tend to be eaten in response to anger or frustration whereas soft, soothing foods, such as ice cream, mashed potatoes and cream cheese, are eaten more as a response to anxiety, sorrow or distress.

unable to recognize them. Next time you open that packet of biscuits, stop and ask yourself what it is you are really feeling. Is it true hunger? If not, what is it you are feeling? Is it hurt, anxiety, fear or anger? Is it sadness or despair? By becoming more in touch with your feelings, you can begin to separate emotional hunger from true hunger. That will help you to control your eating behaviour as you can then learn to eat only in response to your body's natural hunger cues.

Keeping a mood diary can be a big help when you are looking for the link between your triggers and your subsequent feelings. In a mood diary, you record not only the food that you eat but also your feelings when you are eating it and the circumstances that led to them. Were you feeling angry after an argument with your partner? Were you anxious about a meeting tomorrow? Are the foods you are eating at these times different from the foods you normally eat? Try to work back and uncover the chain of events that led to the overeating.

Logging all these details in a diary may seem tedious, but it can be extremely useful in the long run because it will help you identify your triggers and the feelings that they bring about. You can then begin to find ways of managing them that will not lead to weight gain.

2 CHANGE YOUR REACTIONS

As the chain of events leads from triggers to emotions to food, the solution to emotional eating must tackle all three areas. This will involve avoiding the triggers where possible, changing your emotional reactions to them and learning a different coping mechanism. This goes hand-in-hand with healthy eating and limiting your access to high calorie comfort foods at these critical times.

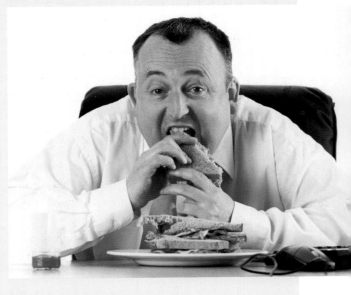

3 MANAGE YOUR TRIGGERS

Whatever your triggers are, you must look at what you can do to avoid them. Seek help and support from friends, family, your work colleagues or other relevant sources. For example, if, like Anne, you are feeling overwhelmed by your responsibilities at home and at work, you should reorganize and delegate household chores, speak to your boss about your workload, and perhaps seek help from social services. Stress is a common cause of emotional eating, and learning to manage it, its sources and its consequences, is essential. Look for practical solutions that you can adhere to in the long term.

4 CHANGE YOUR PERSPECTIVE

The ways in which we react to triggers may be hard to change, because they are often ingrained responses that we learned way back in our childhoods. However, these reactions can be relearned and controlled. You may not always be able to control events, especially those that occurred in your past, but you can at least try to change your emotional reactions to them by using behavioural therapy to change your perspective on them (see pages 114–15). You can also take practical steps to improve your mood, which has a huge effect on your emotional reactions. A positive mood can alter your perception of potential triggers so that they appear less threatening and are less likely to cause you emotional distress.

5 ALTERNATIVE COPING STRATEGIES

Finding an alternative way of coping, when it has always been so much easier to use food, can be challenging and usually involves some degree of trial and error. It may include using relaxation techniques or therapies, or learning to express your feelings, perhaps through art or music, instead of trying to banish them. You may also benefit from joining a support group where you can share your thoughts with, and get advice from, people in similar circumstances to your own. You must find and use whatever works for you, depending on your own individual needs and current lifestyle, no matter how complicated or impractical it may seem to others.

Sometimes, of course, emotional eating stems from more complex psychological issues. If these are at the root of your emotional eating, you should seek professional help in the form of, for example, behavioural counselling, psychotherapy or relationship counselling.

6 CHOOSE YOUR FOOD WISELY

Eating healthy foods and keeping damaging foods at arm's length is the final piece in the jigsaw. When you encounter a particular trigger, your mood at the time, and therefore your reaction to the trigger, may have been influenced by the foods you have been eating. For example, if you are feeling down because your blood sugar levels are low, you will be more sensitive to triggers and your emotional responses to them will be exaggerated.

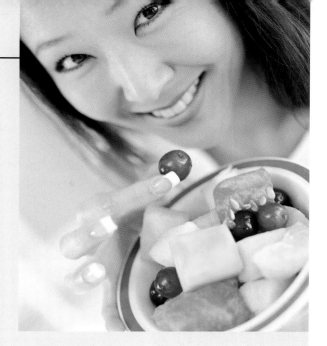

Foods that keep your blood sugar on an even keel, such as slow-release carbohydrates (see pages 52–7), will not only give you sustained energy but also help to improve your mood, making you better able to withstand certain triggers and avoid the emotional roller-coaster that comes from eating inappropriately. Severely restrictive dieting should also be avoided, because consciously depriving yourself of much-loved foods will only increase your desire for them, making you succumb to overeating them when you are under pressure.

PRACTICAL TIPS

In your mind, run through typical scenarios that trigger your emotional eating and rehearse alternative reactions to them so that you are better prepared to face them in the future.

• Challenge your emotions by writing them down and reading them back to yourself. Are they justified? How might another person react? Might there be a hidden reason for these feelings?

• Take positive steps to improve your mood by listening to uplifting music, or enjoying heart-warming films or books.

• Laughter can be the best medicine, and comedy films and humorous books can really help improve your mood and perspective so that you are less likely to overreact to events.

• Do not buy sugary, high-fat snacks or keep them in the house. Stick to healthy snacks only. Then if you really do need to take out your frustrations on something edible you will be forced to take them out on, say, fruit rather than biscuits.

• Accept that learning to change your triggers, your emotional reactions and your behaviour will take time, and that failure is as much a part of the relearning process as is repeated practice.

SEDENTARY LIFESTYLES

In the West, sedentary lifestyles have become the norm for the vast majority of the population, despite the fact that they are known to contribute to short- and long-term weight gain and bring significant health risks. Sedentary living is linked to an increase in mortality similar to that of having diabetes, high blood pressure, or high blood cholesterol and not far behind that associated with smoking. It is linked directly to heart disease and cancer.

In the United Kingdom, for example, two major surveys have found that a third of the adult population takes, on average, less than one 30-minute period of moderate activity per week. Another third takes only irregular bouts of moderate activity, and only 16 percent of men and five percent of women carry out regular moderate activity. In addition, inactivity increases with age.

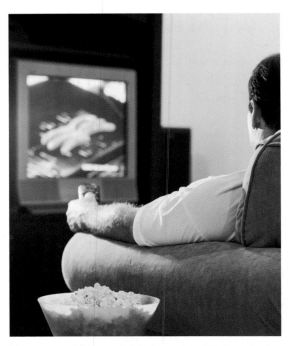

It's so easy to fall into a chair in front of the TV after a hard day's work, but exercise will help you unwind, reducing your stress levels and helping you to relax and, eventually, sleep. You'll even enjoy your food more after a bout of activity.

Other data shows that in all Western countries there has been a general reduction in overall daily energy expenditure, mostly due to modern technology, labour-saving devices and motorized transport. Leisure-time activities have also become more sedentary, and this has all helped to create a large mismatch between the amounts of energy we eat and the amounts we use up. Less than 100 years ago our average daily energy expenditure was around 3000 calories per day, but the average city-dweller now uses less than 1800.

We generally find it difficult to match our calorie intake with our physical activity, because their relationship is asymmetrical. When you reduce your food intake, your body reacts by reducing your metabolic rate to conserve calories. To help this reduction in your metabolic rate, your body tries to limit your physical activity and so you may feel tired, lack energy and motivation, and want to rest. But there is no corresponding urge to increase your physical activity if you eat too much.

THE NEED FOR EXERCISE

As a species, we do not actually have an innate drive to exercise. We dislike exertion and instinctively try to avoid it whenever possible – witness the detours made by people in shopping malls to enter through the one door that is automatic! Our early ancestors were driven to be active by necessity, not desire, in order to obtain food, water and shelter. If you were unable to be active because of genetic disability, illness or injury, you would have perished.

Today, we look after those who are unable to fend for themselves, and we have come to rely more on mental skills than physical agility to obtain our food. The fact remains, however, that our bodies need to be active to remain healthy and to withstand the tendency to gain weight. If necessity no longer drives us to physical activity, we have to make a more conscious decision to take more exercise regularly.

Throughout our history, participation in sport has usually been limited to a relatively small proportion of the population. Nowadays, though, increasing numbers of us are taking part in the many different active leisure pursuits now available, motivated partly by the need to take more exercise and partly by the desire to fill our time. And because, understandably, most of us simply do not enjoy exercise just for the sake of it, we prefer our activities to involve skill or to have additional dimensions, such as camaraderie and team building, bonding and socializing, and excitement and competition.

Walking is exercise requiring no special equipment and can be enjoyed by individuals of all ages. It promotes health in all of them.

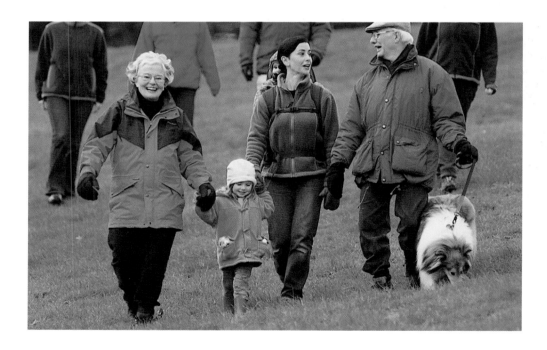

INACTIVITY

When you lead an inactive life, for whatever reason, it's likely that your daily calorie intake will be greater than the amount of calories you burn up every day. The unused calories will end up as body fat, and you will steadily gain weight.

WHAT CAUSES IT?

There are many reasons why we are, on the whole, far less active than we were in years gone by. Occasionally, as in David's case (see below), injury, illness or even a change in personal circumstances may force you to reduce your activity levels quite suddenly and drastically, but more often than not the process is a gradual one.

As technology marches rapidly on, labour-saving devices that remove the need for any physical effort on our part are taking over more and more of our day-to-day activities. Domestic appliances, motor transport, and, increasingly, home entertainment systems and sophisticated electronic communications, have dramatically cut our levels of physical exertion. Few of us have jobs that exercise our bodies as we embrace more cerebral occupations. All of these advances have combined to bring a huge reduction in our average daily energy expenditure.

All this extra time that we are supposedly saving should mean that we have plenty left over in which to take more exercise. Unfortunately, just as technology moves on, so does the pace of our lifestyles and thus, paradoxically, a lack of time is the top reason that people give for not being able to exercise in their leisure time.

Many people join gyms with the best of intentions, then seldom use them because they don't have the time. Others soon get bored with gym-based exercise or are deterred by the ongoing costs of membership. For those that dislike the atmosphere of gyms altogether and prefer to exercise outdoors, poor weather conditions and the relative darkness of the winter months mean that their levels and patterns of activity are inconsistent and irregular across the year.

As well as being a cause of weight gain, inactivity can be a result of it. When you have gained weight for whatever reason you may, like David, become either unable or unwilling to

DAVID came to the clinic having put on a lot of weight over the preceding five years. Once a keen rugby player, cyclist and mountaineer, he had gained the weight during a prolonged period of forced rest while recovering from a back injury. After that, he had never managed to return to his previous level of physical activity because of his excess weight, and had replaced his active outdoor lifestyle with more sedentary indoor pursuits, often revolving around food and alcohol. As a result, his intake of both had increased significantly and his weight appeared to be climbing relentlessly year after year. He was unhappy about this, because being overweight was slowly eroding his confidence and increasing his tendency to drink.

exercise, perhaps out of pain or for fear of aggravating or repeating the injury. Some people simply claim that they do not like exercise, but usually the problem is that they have developed a psychological resistance to it over the years. If you dislike the idea of exercise, perhaps you have an inaccurate picture in your mind of what it actually entails or have tried it before and found it painful or otherwise unpleasant. Maybe you have become disillusioned with exercise because you have failed to achieve your goals.

If you have never exercised in your adult life, it could be because you just don't see yourself as the exercising type. Or maybe you dislike the idea of becoming hot and sweaty, or feel awkward and ridiculous at the thought of putting on trainers and walking, for all intents and purposes, aimlessly. If you were labelled 'bad at sport' at school, then perhaps you are harboring uncertainties about your sporting abilities that stem from your childhood. All or any of these barriers may be holding you back from taking part in sports or other forms of exercise.

THE CONSEQUENCES

People tend not to be very good at cutting down on their food intake to match any reduction in energy expenditure, so when you become less active you often carry on eating as you always have. This creates a mismatch between your energy intake and your energy output and so you gain weight.

A further problem is that your under-used muscles tend to shrink. Muscle tissue burns up more calories than fat tissue, even when you are resting. The loss of muscle that comes from inactivity means that not only are you burning fewer calories than if you were active but you are also burning fewer calories when your body is resting.

As David discovered (see opposite page), inactivity can lead to weight gain, which makes you even less active, leading to more weight gain. The gradual reduction in activity may occur very slowly and be so subtle that you are not even aware of it, but over a period of years, even if you are not eating more food, you find your weight just keeps going up and up.

The process will naturally be accelerated if less activity is also accompanied, as in David's case, by greater food intake. Eating often fills the void previously occupied by activity. An increase in size can also lead to more emotional eating and drinking if it creates uncomfortable feelings and poor self-esteem.

Reversing this cycle by combining increased activity with a reduction in calorie intake was an essential part of David's weight-loss programme. Few dieters have been able to maintain their weight loss long term without increasing their activity levels.

Inactivity Recovery Programme

1 FIRST STEPS

Many people automatically assume that exercise inevitably involves something gruelling, such as regular five-lap jogs around the local park. They have somehow come to associate exercise with pain and duress and so are totally resistant to the very idea of it. But strenuous exercise is not necessarily what you need to help you to lose weight.

If you have never exercised formally before, and dislike the thought of launching yourself into a structured exercise programme, you can start by simply reducing the amount of time you spend sitting around, and incorporating small amounts of extra physical activity into your day. At work, this could involve spending less time sitting at your desk and actually delivering notes, memos or letters by hand rather than using email or the phone. Take breaks every 30 minutes and walk around: go for a drink of water or just to stretch your legs. Use the stairs instead of the lift.

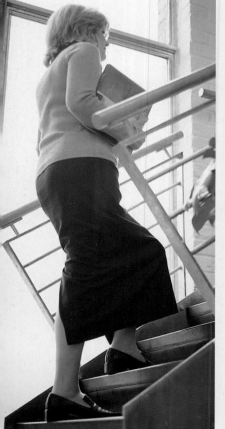

In the home, the most common sedentary activities are watching TV, playing computer games and using the internet, so limit the amount of time you give to these activities. Watching less television also means you are less likely to reach for snacks as well. Look for other, more useful and active things that you could do instead, such as gardening, housework or preparing and cooking interesting meals. When you do watch TV, give up the remote control or put it in a central place, out of your immediate reach, so that you have to get up out of your seat every time you want to change channels.

You can increase your range of activity opportunities in many other easy ways: park farther away from the supermarket entrance and carry the shopping to your car instead of using a trolley; get off the bus one or two stops earlier than usual and walk the rest of the way.

All these activities are forms of exercise that you can simply build into your daily life, and, unlike jogging or going to the gym, you don't need to set aside any specific time for them. They need no specialist equipment or training, cost little or nothing in terms of time or money, and can all add up to a significant contribution to your daily energy expenditure.

2 LEISURE ACTIVITIES

As well as adding opportunistic exercise to your daily routine, you may be able to put time aside for more regular periods of leisure-time activity. Again, this need not be punishing or involve hours spent in a gym but can include everyday exercise such as walking or cycling to the shops, or social activities such as dancing, bowling, or tennis. These can get you out and about and are especially good for building up your confidence if you have not exercised previously. Many gyms now run an assortment of classes that suit every taste and level, from yoga to Pilates and belly-dancing to boxing, so you can choose to exercise alone, in a group, or with a friend for support and encouragement.

3 STRUCTURED EXERCISE PROGRAMMES

If, as well as losing weight, you want to change your body shape or improve specific aspects of your health, such as heart and lung function, then you need a more structured exercise programme. This will usually involve a combination of aerobic cardiovascular exercise and resistance training involving lifting weights (see pages 140–49). You don't necessarily need a personal trainer, but hiring one is a good investment for motivation, especially at the beginning.

4 EVALUATE YOUR GOALS AND EXPECTATIONS

Attainable goals and expectations are as relevant to exercise as they are to weight loss. You must have a realistic idea of the ability of exercise to burn up calories, and of the extent to which it can help you lose weight. If not, you may find that you overcompensate for exercise with excessive food intake. This is especially true of women, who tend to view exercise more as a punishment and so reward themselves with a slice of cake afterwards.

Exercise can only help you to lose fat if your calorie intake remains static, and even then, results are not immediate. Always think of exercise as a great benefit to your overall health, rather than just as a means to weight loss. That way you are less likely to feel disappointed and give up if the weight is not coming off as fast as you would like.

It is equally important to set realistic goals for the type and level of activity you want to undertake, because failing to achieve unrealistic aims may also lead to disappointment and abandonment of the exercise programme. You must begin with small changes that you can build on. If you set tough, unachievable, or

THE PSYCHOLOGICAL BENEFITS OF EXERCISE

The benefits of exercise during weight loss include more than just an increase in calorie expenditure. Exercise also provides psychological benefits with the release of feel-good brain chemicals that increase your overall sense of well-being, lift your mood and improve your self-confidence and self-esteem, all of which are associated with reduced anxiety and depression. Exercise is also a great stress-buster and will help you to sleep more soundly.

unsustainable goals, you will soon become demotivated. Also bear in mind that inappropriately intensive exercise may actually be counterproductive because it can increase your appetite (see pages 48–51), so you must be clear about your objectives and set goals that you can maintain in the long term.

5 MAINTAINING MOTIVATION

The best way to maintain your motivation is to choose an exercise activity that you enjoy. This is the only way to sustain your enthusiasm on those cold, damp winter evenings. It is also a good idea to change your exercise routine regularly, again to prevent you from becoming bored. Always working through the same exercises can become monotonous. Even small changes can help, such as altering the route you normally walk or cycle along or performing exercises in a different order. Better still, if your motivation starts to flag, take up a new activity that challenges your mind as well as your body. Try to maintain variety.

Keeping your exercise programme flexible is also important. If you cannot run outdoors because of bad weather, then swim indoors, or if you lack time one day, just build exercise around your errands. Do what you can on the day and get away from the brittle 'all-or-nothing' thinking that can often lead people to abandoning exercise altogether.

6 BREAKING PSYCHOLOGICAL BARRIERS

You can overcome any psychological issues that are holding you back by building up your exercise activities gradually. Start very slowly by taking up a leisurely form of exercise such as walking in the park. If you enjoy swimming but lack self-confidence, then try to go when the pool is less likely to be full. To build up your confidence, begin with exercise you can do at home before venturing outside, for instance follow the routines of an exercise video or work out with light weights or an exercise cycle.

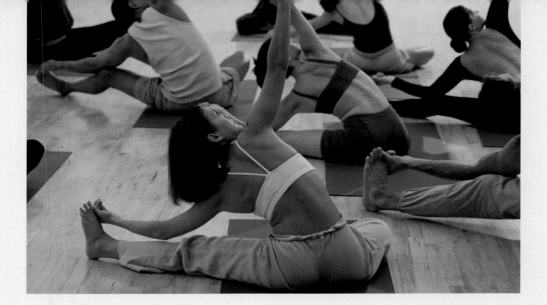

Breaking through psychological barriers also involves shedding any misconceptions and prejudices about exercise, body shape and age. You can be active at any size and at any age. All of us have to begin from the level we at are today, and it is never too late to start.

7 DIETARY CHANGES

Exercise, especially when carried out regularly, is very good for the prevention of weight gain. But if your aim is to lose weight, then exercise alone will rarely do the trick if not accompanied by appropriate changes to your diet. A sensible diet can prevent you from overeating and thus negating the benefits you are gaining from exercise.

PRACTICAL TIPS

Remember that any activity is better than no activity. Doing a little every day is better than occasional bouts of severe exercise, which may lead to injury.

• Exercise with a friend for fun, psychological support and motivation.
• If you spend your evenings watching television, take up knitting or a similar hobby that you can do at the same time. This will help you to keep burning those calories and to avoid snacking.
• Being active most of the time throughout the day is better than being inactive all day and then exercising vigorously for 30 minutes.
• Take up domestic hobbies that involve some physical effort, such as gardening or decorating – even dusting and vacuuming can help you burn more calories, especially if you do them with gusto.

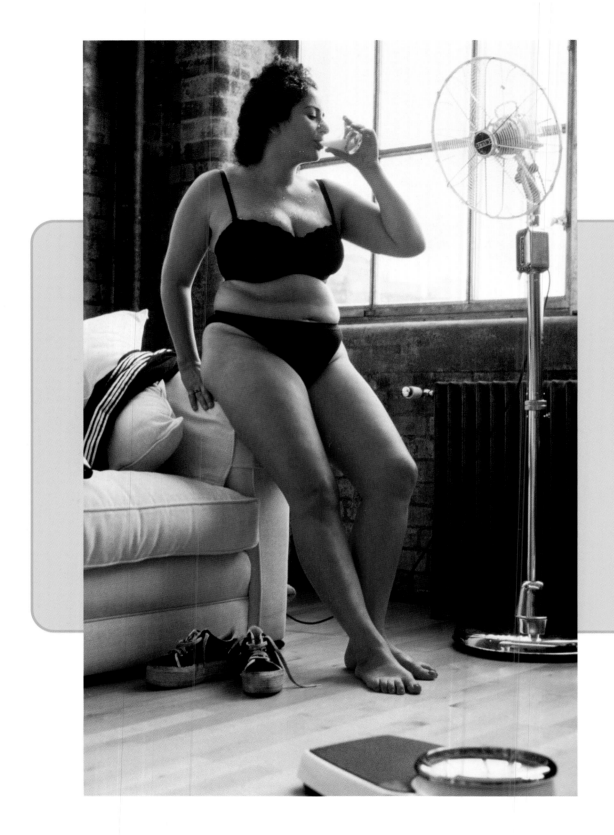

4

HOW TO CONTROL YOUR WEIGHT

THE EVIDENCE FOR DIETS

If you want to lose weight, finding an effective diet plan can be extremely difficult. There are so many to choose from, and new plans appear as often as new trends in fashion and tend to last about as long. Most of them will help you to lose weight, but few will provide what you really need, which is true long-term weight loss. All commercial diet plans, new and old, back their claims with supposedly scientific evidence, often coupled with endorsements from satisfied customers (who may or may not exist) and frequently from minor celebrities who need the money.

As far as the scientific evidence is concerned, you should always be sceptical about the claims of commercial diets, and even the noncommercial products – diet plans formulated by nutritionists and dietitians concerned with promoting health rather than making a profit – are not definitive. They are based on the latest information about nutrition, health and weight, but are constantly being refined and revised as as scientific knowledge advances.

This is because our present understanding of the human body is not complete, and research results can be misleading and open to misinterpretation. The best evidence comes from looking at diet and health trends around the world, observing the eating behaviour of people who have successfully lost weight in the long term, and applying our growing knowledge of nutrition and physiology based on cumulative scientific research.

A DIET THAT WORKS

Scientists must be careful how they evaluate and interpret their research data, because any flaws in it may lead them to inaccurate conclusions and most long-term studies on weight cannot, unfortunately, be performed under perfectly controlled conditions that will allow flawless results. They have to rely mostly on honest and accurate reporting from a usually small number of participants, members of the public who won't always be able to comply with the strict rules of the study. This is especially true of commercial and prescriptive diets, because some are easier to stick to than others over a long period of time.

Despite these uncertainties, some reliable conclusions have emerged time and again from numerous international research studies. Of these, one of the most important is the correlation between a high intake of animal proteins and fat and an increased risk of heart disease and some cancers. Conversely, increasing the consumption of protein and unsaturated fats derived from fish and plant sources, and dietary fibre from whole grains, fruit and vegetables that are also high in antioxidants, appears to confer protection.

Many of these conclusions form the basis of the dietary guidelines set out later in this chapter. These guidelines, when combined with other healthy lifestyle factors, have been overwhelmingly endorsed by people who have successfully lost a substantial amount of weight and been able to maintain their weight loss over the long term. According to research, this diet is also superior to a simple calorie-controlled diet. It is the diet that almost 95 percent of Americans who have achieved long-term weight loss claim to have used, so it has been shown to work for real people in real-life situations. It is also supported by our current scientific knowledge of appetite regulation and energy balance in the body, which provides the theoretical basis for how such a diet might work.

THE ROLE OF LEPTIN

Some of the latest dietary research to emerge from leading US universities has centred on the role of a hormone, leptin. The results of this research provide further proof for some of the theories already discussed in this book.

Leptin, which is made by fat cells in the body, is not a newly discovered hormone but its actions within the body have, until now, been unclear. It seems to act on the appetite centre in the brain to reduce appetite. The levels of the hormone normally increase in proportion to the amount of body fat, so the more fat you have, the higher your leptin levels. What had confused clinicians until now was why, if leptin acts on the brain to reduce appetite, do overweight people still have such strong appetites despite having higher levels of circulating leptin?

The answer is that the appetite centre can become less sensitive to leptin, and

THE UNHEALTHY WESTERN DIET

The average Western diet is high in saturated fats and refined sugar compared to the average Japanese diet. This includes more mono-and polyunsaturated fats, such as soya and vegetables oils, and much less sugar. The link between diet and disease is clear; many 'Western' diseases are much rarer in Japan.

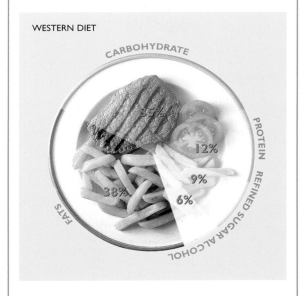

WESTERN DIET

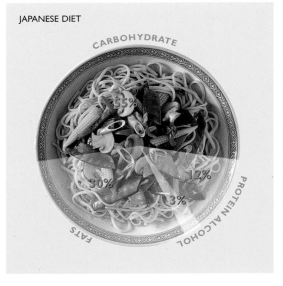

JAPANESE DIET

some people become increasingly resistant its effects. Leptin resistance can occur spontaneously or with ageing, or as a result of repeated cycles of dieting and weight fluctuation that result in fluctuations in leptin levels. People with leptin resistance require more of the hormone to have the same effect on their appetite, which, in turn, means they require an increasingly greater fat mass to produce it. In other words, they need more body fat in order to produce

LEPTIN INJECTIONS FIGHT GENETIC OBESITY

Individuals with a rare genetic disorder preventing their fat cells from producing leptin have insatiable appetites and become morbidly obese as young children. Giving them injections of leptin appears to reduce their appetite, allowing them to lose weight.

SOME DIFFERENT DIETS

Name and description	Disadvantages	Advantages
Low-fat diet	You exclude or limit foods that are particularly rich in fat such as fried food, many types of meat, condiments, dairy products and dressings. 'Low fat' can also mean 'low taste', as the palatability of many low-fat products is affected.	Reducing fat intake can help to reduce the risk of heart disease. It is easy to maintain as the starchier foods and fruits and vegetables, which are the bulk of your consumption, are very filling.
High-fibre diet	You eat a large amount of fruits, vegetables, cereals, nuts and wholefoods at the expense of fattier foods. Too much fibre can produce side effects such as flatulence and diarrhoea and interfere with the absorption of minerals.	Fibre in the form of cereals, legumes, fruits and vegetables can help to reduce the risk of some kinds of cancer, particularly colon cancer, and also helps to prevent other gut problems.
Hay diet	You eat a lot of vegetables, salads and fruits and restrict concentrated sources of proteins, carbohydrates and fats. Potatoes and pastas must not be eaten in the same meal as meat and dairy.	If you do restrict the amount of fat and calories then you will lose weight. The diet also encourages eating more fruits and vegetables.
The Atkins Diet	You can eat all the meat, cheese, eggs and fat you want while limiting the type and amount of carbohydrates. Low-carbohydrate high-protein diets can exceed recommended quantities of cholesterol, fat, saturated fat and protein. They don't sustain your nutritional needs.	You will lose weight and don't have to count calories or adjust portion size.

enough leptin to adequately suppress their hunger, so their appetite control system leans towards greater body fat accumulation.

The actions of leptin can also explain why it can be so hard to maintain weight loss. When you lose body fat, your leptin levels go down. The suppressing effect of leptin on your appetite is therefore reduced, and so your appetite may begin to increase if you lose too much body fat. Your body tries to restore its fat reserves to what it considers to be a more desirable level, even if it is not aesthetically pleasing. The researchers also found that a high-fat diet appears to reduce leptin levels whereas a high carbohydrate (whole grain), low-fat diet boosts leptin levels and therefore helps to reduce appetite. Exercise may also help to improve leptin sensitivity.

The research on leptin confirms that your appetite and your weight are to an important extent determined by your genes, and that repeated cycles of fat loss and fat gain can be damaging to your physiology and lead to weight gain in the long run. It also shows that weight maintenance is a lifelong process that requires a similarly long-term approach, and that a low-fat, high-carbohydrate diet is the most appropriate regime for helping to control appetite.

CHOOSING AN EFFECTIVE DIET PLAN

When considering any diet plan, you should seek answers to the following questions:

- How reliable are the scientific claims and evidence behind the diet? If a diet sounds too good to be true, it almost always is.
- Does the diet have any short- or long-term implications for your health?
- How practical is the diet?
- How flexible is it?
- What is the financial cost? You may have to rely on specific products as part of the diet.
- If the diet is very restrictive or complex, what will it cost you in terms of time, effects on your social life and changes to your lifestyle? Can you bear these costs for very long?
- Does it teach the nutritional skills required for managing your weight for life?
- Apart from helping you to lose weight, is the diet also likely to be of long-term benefit to your health and well-being?

These are all important points to consider if you want a diet plan that is going to help you control your appetite, lose and maintain your weight, improve your health and end the cycle of yo-yo dieting.

ARE YOU READY TO CHANGE?

Knowing how your body handles its energy intake and expenditure gives you a valuable insight into the physical aspects of dieting, but knowledge alone is not enough to ensure lasting weight-loss success. You also need skills that will help you to change your behaviour, so that you can make and stick to the lifestyle changes that will help you lose weight and improve your overall health.

Acquiring these skills is a form of behavioural therapy. In this case, it is the process of shedding unfavourable eating and lifestyle habits, and learning and reinforcing favourable patterns of behaviour until they become routine. It will make you aware of negative patterns of thinking and aspects of your present lifestyle that may be causing or perpetuating weight gain and stopping you from losing weight.

Changing your behaviour is a slow process, however, and it usually happens in a number of distinct stages as shown in the diagram below. Try to identify where you are in this cycle, and don't try to change your behaviour unless you really are ready to do so. If you're not, you are more likely to give up or fail.

Before you start trying to modify your behaviour, though, ask yourself the following questions so that you are clear in your own mind how far you are prepared to change the way you live:

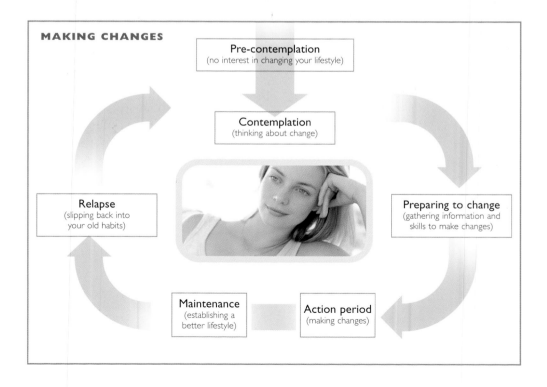

MAKING CHANGES

Pre-contemplation
(no interest in changing your lifestyle)

Contemplation
(thinking about change)

Relapse
(slipping back into your old habits)

Preparing to change
(gathering information and skills to make changes)

Maintenance
(establishing a better lifestyle)

Action period
(making changes)

- Firstly, what is your goal of weight loss actually worth to you? What would it do for you? How might it change your life? Are you doing this for yourself or to please someone else?
- Is your goal realistic? Can you really achieve it if you want it enough? Are you prepared to make the sacrifices and do the work that will inevitably be involved?
- Where does losing weight rank in your list of priorities for your life?
- Are there any obstacles, physical or emotional, that may prevent you from making the changes that you want? Does any part of you, conscious or subconscious, object to change and if so, why?
- Is your goal in keeping with your values and beliefs? Are you biased against overweight people? Perhaps that is why you do not want to be one?
- If you do change your lifestyle and behaviour, will that affect anyone else, such as your partner or children? Might they object? You may need their support in order to make your changes workable and permanent.

The answers to these questions often reveal the reasons behind unsuccessful attempts at changing behaviour and losing weight. By asking them before you start, you can often alert yourself to any problems that might crop up later and prevent you from succeeding. And if you find that you are having difficulty sticking to changes that you've made, return to these questions to help you pinpoint and deal with the cause of the problem.

Finally, you have to accept that unless your weight gain was caused by ill health, it was your own negative eating habits and lifestyle that led to it and so you must accept responsibility for it. Then you must recognize that the changes needed to achieve your goal will ultimately have to come from you and be maintained by you. You need to be solely responsible and apply the resources within you. You cannot rely on anyone or anything else.

People who remain in denial about the extent of their negative lifestyle and eating behaviour are less likely to be proactive in losing weight, and often lack the motivation to make or maintain changes to their diet or lifestyle. Such people are more likely to search for reasons other than themselves to blame for their situation, and therefore more likely to seek quick-fix solutions or miracle diets in the futile hope that they will produce effortless, lasting weight loss.

MOTIVATION AND EXPECTATIONS

Losing weight takes time, and may involve some uncomfortable changes to your lifestyle. So to maintain your enthusiasm to succeed, you need good incentives and motivation – in particular, the right kind of motivation.

CULTURAL INFLUENCES

Ideally, an individual's incentive to lose weight should be better physical and mental health, but more often people just want to look good and feel better about themselves. They imagine their lives will be instantly transformed by weight loss, and picture themselves as becoming happy, successful people. When these expectations are not met, as so often happens, they simply stop trying.

Contemporary culture plays an important role in setting such improbable expectations by giving us slender role models so that we associate being thin with prestige, success, love and happiness. On television and in film, overweight women tend to play parts such as homely mothers or unhappy singles, while the overwhelming majority of glamorous female heroines are slim if not thin, and magazines continually bombard us with articles on weight loss as we peer at models that are becoming increasingly thinner.

As a result, many women set their expectations of what is desirable at similar levels and feel compelled to achieve them, forgetting that they are unnatural and perhaps unattainable without risk to their health – quite a few celebrities have unhealthy eating habits or use drugs and cigarettes to maintain their weight. Many have surgery to achieve perfection or create a body of unnatural proportions, and often have their own cooks and stylists or spend hours in the gym with their personal

Media images that equate slimness with success lead many women to set their expectations of what is desirable at unrealistic levels.

trainers. Even then, it can take hours of make-up and hair styling, plus careful lighting and computer enhancement, to produce the images of them that we see.

We are led to believe that we can, and perhaps should, aspire to look like celebrities and models so that we too can be happy, attractive and lovable. When we do not measure up to these ideals, we feel inadequate and so want to lose weight, but this kind of motivation is one that is very likely to lead to disappointment and can can damage our self-esteem and body image.

BODY IMAGE

In a recent survey of British women, 75 percent thought they were fat, 89 percent wanted to lose weight and 95 percent had dieted at some time. A staggering 15 percent said they would be willing to give up five years of their life in exchange for the ability to reach their ideal weight. These findings reflect increasing levels of clinical and subclinical eating disorders among younger women in the West, and globally where Western imagery and ideology has permeated through, but culture is only one factor that contributes to body image.

Your body image is the mental picture you have of your physical self and your emotional reaction to it, be it positive or negative. It can change from day to day or even after a big meal. It can be affected by your mood, by seeing the wrong number on the bathroom scales, seeing an unflattering photograph of yourself or hearing a critical comment. Family, friends and partners can shape your body image throughout your life.

Because many women define themselves by their physical appearance and weight, they use weight control as a tool to improve their self-worth. They tend to punish themselves for not having the perfect body, for instance by not allowing themselves to buy new clothes or go on holiday until they have lost weight. Until then, love, life and enjoyment is put on hold.

Unfortunately, investing your happiness in your body size is risky because weight loss to improve self-esteem rarely works, and certainly does not last. It remains a quick-fix answer to a much deeper problem and is likely to lead to disappointment when unrealistic expectations are not met. To lose weight long term, you have to begin by dissociating self-esteem from weight and appearance, because there is a limit to how much you can control your body shape and weight without risking your mental and physical health.

SKINNY MODELS SET A BAD EXAMPLE

In one study, a group of women were given some women's magazines to read. Almost three-quarters of them reported feeling worse about their looks after reading the magazines, even though the models pictured in them were 13–19 percent thinner than would be healthy for their height.

Your body shape naturally changes with time, and you may never again be the same weight, nor should you try to be, as when you were 21. You can learn to love yourself and your body no matter what size and shape you are. The process involves learning self-acceptance and a degree of fat acceptance, despite the current cultural ideals. You have to challenge your own prejudices about fat and favourable traits such as competence, desirability, entitlement and happiness, and immunize yourself against cultural stereotypes and bias. Doing this successfully will also encourage you to take part in social and physical activities you may have avoided out of embarrassment about your body size.

For successful long-term weight loss, your motivation should be that you want to improve your quality of life, not that you want to enhance your self-esteem. Losing weight should be a way of being kinder to and respecting yourself and of taking better care of yourself and your body. You should aim to be healthier and fitter and to increase your chances of living a longer and fuller life. Most importantly, you must want to do it for yourself and not to please other people.

Think of losing weight by learning to eat more healthily as an extension of your self-respect. By taking a more positive frame of mind, you are more likely to enjoy the process of losing weight by seeing it as a way of caring for yourself, rather than as a process of deprivation and a painful means to an end.

REALISTIC EXPECTATIONS

When you ask women how much weight they want to lose, most say 30 percent of their body weight. They would feel dissatisfied with losing 20 percent, and often see losing only 15 percent as a failure of the diet. When most studies show that under two percent of people are able to achieve and maintain their ideal body weight long term, you can see the huge gap between expectations and what is achievable. A 20 percent drop in body weight requires an almost identical percentage reduction in long-term calorie intake, and a 30 percent drop calls for a 30 percent reduction, which is difficult to achieve in a short time and even harder to maintain in the long run.

It is better, therefore, to aim for a realistic compromise between perfection and absolute failure. Women who have greater self-acceptance and set more realistic goals (see pages 122–3) have greater self-esteem and, paradoxically, a greater overall sense of control in their lives. Failing repeatedly to achieve

CHILDHOOD INFLUENCES AFFECT SELF-IMAGE

Children raised in families that nurture body-shape acceptance at any weight are more likely to have a positive body image and greater self-esteem that is unrelated to weight. On the other hand, derogatory comments and a negative view of obesity in childhood generate poorer self-image in later life.

perfection only reinforces low confidence and poor self-esteem, and creates a sense of failure. It can be draining and takes energy away from other, more important areas of your life. It is far better to lose a reasonable amount of weight and stabilize yourself comfortably at that lower level than to end up yo-yo dieting.

You also need to be realistic about the changes that losing weight will bring about in your life. Having made the decision to lose weight, you may initially feel empowered and start making sudden and drastic changes to other aspects of your life. This is far too ambitious, because it's unreasonable to make lots of changes in a short time and then expect to maintain them. Although it may be manageable at first, when your new expectations fail to materialize you are likely to give up both on them and on losing weight. You must not expect your life and the world around you to change overnight just because you are on a diet. Lifestyles, behaviours and attitudes are formed over many years and take a long time to change.

Setting yourself realistic, achievable goals for changing your behaviour and lifestyle is more likely to keep you

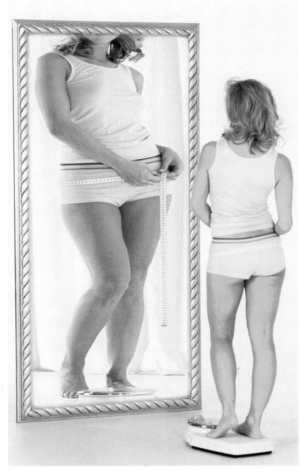

There can be a big difference between your body image and reality. A negative body image can often involve the mistaken belief that you are badly overweight.

motivated to lose weight – and if you lack motivation, you will have to make up for it with a lot of willpower! If you make eating a healthier diet and taking part in more physical activities your goal, then lasting weight loss will inevitably follow when you attain it.

KEEPING A FOOD DIARY

Before you can start to change your eating habits, you need to get a clear idea of exactly what they are, and one of the best ways to do this is to keep a food diary. Get a large diary with plenty of room for each day's entries, and record in it exactly what and how much you eat.

Enter the information immediately after each meal or snack, in as much detail as possible while it is still fresh in your mind, and include details of everything you drink so that you get as complete a picture as possible of your daily calorie intake. Noting your mood, the setting, the time, and events immediately prior to and after eating can also be helpful, as can details of your physical activities, although it might be easier to keep a separate diary for monitoring these.

FOOD DIARY

You can adjust the template, below, to suit your needs. Make sure you enter any snacks and drinks. It can also help to give a rating of 1 and 10 according to how hungry you were for each meal. For example, 2 could represent not really hungry, 9 could be very hungry.

	Breakfast	Mid-morning	Lunch	Mid-afternoon	Dinner	Mood/feelings before/after eating
Monday						
Tuesday						
Wednesday						
Thursday						
Friday						
Saturday						
Sunday						

Many people find the idea of keeping a food diary absurd and tedious and cannot see the benefit, but the very act of keeping a diary can itself help you reduce food intake by simply making you more aware of what you are eating. It can also help you to identify your problem foods, your negative eating patterns and your triggers to overeating so that you can set goals for improvement. It is easier to find your problem if you have the evidence written down in front of you. A diary can also help you to monitor changes and to target problems as they occur, but you should monitor your weight no more than once a week, if at all. You can tell from your clothes if you are losing inches.

STIMULUS CONTROL

Another benefit of keeping a food diary is that it can highlight circumstances or external cues that are making you overeat or snack. Perhaps it is the sight of certain foods, or watching TV, or going out for a meal that triggers your overeating, or maybe it's a response to an emotional cue such as anger or sorrow, a result of drinking alcohol, or a way of filling time when you're bored.

Once you've identified specific events or circumstances that prompt you to overeat, you can then try to avoid those triggers or devise better ways of coping with them. If it is the smell of freshly cooked bread in the supermarket then sets you off, head straight for the fresh produce when you enter the store, or shop only when you are full. If the biscuit tin is the trigger then keep it out of sight – out of sight and out of mind!

Some people find that they are 'all or nothing' when it comes to certain foods. For instance, if they have one biscuit, they have to have finish the packet, but they seem to cope better with the idea of having none at all than having a small portion. If you are one of these people, you may have to ban such foods from the house altogether.

LEARNING SELF-CONTROL

Some triggers are impossible to avoid completely, so you will have to learn to control your responses to them. This means exposing yourself to your problem situations and trying to change your reactions. You may initially have a heightened urge to eat, but this usually subsides within the next five to thirty minutes and the challenge is to generate thoughts that motivate you and that will help to quell your eating urge during that time.

When faced with tempting but calorie-laden food, remind yourself how damaging it will be to your health and to your body. Visualize the look and feel of excess fat, then picture yourself at the weight you want to be and imagine how wonderful you will feel then. Alternatively, remind yourself that for the calories in one mouthful of a sugary, high-fat food you could eat a plateful of healthier alternatives, then think about how much more filling that would be and how much better for your health, your skin and your vitality. You can practise such tactics in advance so that they become your natural patterns of thinking.

Changing your responses to overeating triggers is a relearning process that must be reinforced with repetition, and if you fail at it to start with – as many people do – just keep trying and eventually you will succeed. Begin with situations where you already feel confident and in control and go from there. Try what works for you, and proceed at your own pace.

Recognizing the trigger factors that cause you to 'go crazy' with food is the first step in controlling them. Many people are completely unaware of how much they eat in a day – and why.

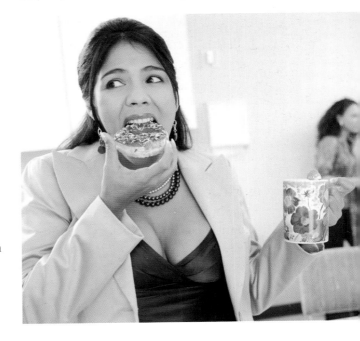

SETTING GOALS

The best way to reach your ultimate objective of successful, long-term weight loss is to set yourself a series of short-term goals that will act as stepping stones to get you there. It is vital to get these short-term goals right, because if you choose them well they can be incredibly motivating, but poorly judged goals can lead to failure and disappointment.

Firstly, concentrate on setting small short-term goals that are reasonable and genuinely within your capacity and don't call for major changes in your present lifestyle. These could include, for example, cutting out sugary snacks and getting into the habit of walking for at least 20 minutes a day. Once you have successfully accomplished and maintained these, then set your next short-term goals, for instance to eat more fruit and vegetables and take up swimming. Avoid setting yourself over-ambitious goals that need drastic changes in your lifestyle. These changes may seem easy to make when you feel very motivated at the beginning but, as often happens, you may not be able to maintain them.

Secondly, concentrate on your short-term goals rather than on your ultimate target of a lasting reduction in your weight. When you achieve these goals, the resulting changes in your behaviour – such as walking for longer, limiting alcohol, cutting out fried foods and eating more vegetables – will automatically lead to weight loss. It is also a good idea to devise several pathways to each goal so that if one becomes blocked, you can change to an alternative route, and the multiple natures of your goals and pathways will help you to stay motivated.

A lot of unhappiness comes from setting one rigid and over-ambitious target and then pursuing it self-destructively, no matter how unsatisfying the journey or unreachable the final destination. On the other hand, achieving lots of little successes can be motivating and empowering because they will give you a sense of progress and increase your self-confidence, inspiring you to set more and more short-term goals that eventually result in your long-term goal.

SELF REINFORCEMENT

You may find that giving yourself a small reward for achieving a goal keeps you motivated and helps to reinforce new behaviours. Just be careful not to make the reward the incentive for changing your behaviour. The reward must remain just that, a gesture of self-acknowledgement for achieving a goal, and ideally it should not consist of food that you are trying to cut down on or give up.

AVOID SETTING WEIGHT-LOSS TARGETS

When you set targets for weight, all of your sense of achievement literally hangs in the balance each time you step on the scales. The 'wrong' number may leave you with a real sense of demoralization even though you may have made good progress in changing your behaviour. It takes time for the changes in your behaviour to be reflected in changes in your weight, so keep your focus on changing your behaviour.

However, if you feel that you really do have to set yourself weight-loss targets, then aim for no more than a five percent reduction in your body weight at any one time. Once you have reached and maintained that, you can aim for your next five percent reduction.

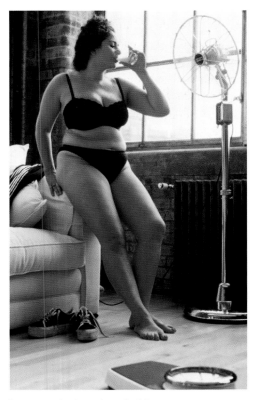

Losing weight depends on building on your successes. If you are successful in a lot of small ways you will ultimately be successful in your larger goals.

GUIDELINES FOR GOAL-SETTING

When you frame your goals in your mind, focus on the pluses and challenge the minuses:

- **Be Positive.** Instead of thinking 'I hate my body!' or 'I don't want to be fat!', make your thoughts more positive – 'I want to feel great!' or 'I want to look healthier!' Similarly, instead of 'I mustn't have any biscuits', think instead 'I must have some fruit'. Aim for the positive and avoid the negative.
- **Be Detailed.** Think through what you want to achieve and how you will feel and look. Visualize yourself as you would like to be, doing the things you want to be doing. Do this on a regular basis to reinforce these ideals and make them feel real and within your reach.
- **Be Realistic.** Try to set attainable goals and be realistic in your expectations of how your life may change. Don't imagine that the world will suddenly change because you have lost weight – this will only set you up for disappointment.
- **Be Clear.** Keep your goals simple by setting small criteria for changing your behaviour. One change or goal for the week may be enough if that is what is manageable for you. If you are failing with one goal, then re-evaluate it or shift your focus to another one.
- **Be Prepared.** Attaining your goals will involve making some sacrifices, so think carefully about the things that you are genuinely willing to give up and those you are not.

STRATEGIES FOR SUCCESS

Why do some people succeed at losing weight long term while others habitually fail? The answer is not greater willpower but the attitudes, beliefs and mental strategies that they use to overcome psychological barriers – there are rarely any physical barriers that prevent people from losing weight. Destructive patterns of thinking that compromise their motivation and their beliefs in their own abilities are what prevent people from achieving their targets. The good news is that as well as learning to do things differently, we can learn to think differently.

CHANGING YOUR PERSPECTIVES

If you want to change your behaviour, you first have to change your perspectives – the ways in which you view and react to events. Remember, though, that your thought patterns and perspectives are a deep and integral part of who you are. They have been reinforced over your lifetime and are deeply embedded in your psyche. Updating your perspectives (see box on page 127) takes time, but it can dramatically improve the way in which you approach difficult situations. It will help you to remain positive and resilient in the face of perceived disappointment, and make you more likely to succeed.

IMPROVING YOUR MOOD

Your state of mind can affect your perspectives and behaviour, so when you are in a negative mood you tend to become irritated, despondent and more likely to give up. Try to become more aware of your moods and learn to be more proactive in steering them in a positive direction. This will allow you to challenge negative thoughts and beliefs that may have prevented you from accomplishing your goals in the past.

When you feel down, think of activities and experiences that lift your mood, such as listening to uplifting music, wearing colourful clothing, reading a funny book, watching an upbeat, feel-good film or laughing with friends. Some people write down inspirational or motivational anecdotes, sayings or quotes on pieces of paper. Then they stick them in strategic positions, such as on the biscuit tin or the bathroom mirror, so that reading them maintains their positivity, motivation and enthusiasm. Use whatever works for you.

IMPROVING YOUR BODY IMAGE

It is worth stressing that improving your body image is an important part of behavioural therapy for weight loss. Many people are driven by negative emotions such as low self-esteem, inadequacy, a need to prove themselves or a need to feel accepted and loved. Unfortunately, more often than not they fail to find fulfilment in their achievements until they confront and work through the causes of these sometimes destructive emotions.

SEROTONIN

One of the 'Big Three' neurotransmitters — the others being dopamine and noradrenaline, serotonin plays a central role in many brain functions. Scientists refer to it as 'the body's happy chemical' because low levels result in depression and moodiness. As well as being central to a wide range of normal brain functions, such as sleep, ageing, eating patterns, biorhythms and pain perception, it is also involved with abnormal mental conditions such as anxiety, stress, eating disorders and addictions. A fundamental mechanism of antidepressant action is to increase serotonin in the brain. In particular, the selective serotonin reuptake inhibitor (SSRI) class of antidepressants includes some of the most commonly prescribed drugs on the planet such as Zoloft, Prozac and Seroxat.

The brain has to make its own serotonin by converting the amino acid, tryptophan. Virtually all of our tryptophan comes from the diet, and so eating foods that are rich in tryptophan can boost serotonin levels and ease the symptoms of depression. Good sources include turkey, milk, cottage cheese, nuts, sunflower seeds, peas, beans, bananas, fish and eggs. Carbohydrate foods can facilitate the brain's uptake of tryptophan. The best ones are salad leaves, oats, barley, apples, pears, grapes and other fruits.

The pursuit of perfection as a way of increasing self-esteem is misguided, but learning self-acceptance and dissociating your appearance from your self-esteem can be liberating. In essence, it is learning to love yourself, being kinder and less critical of yourself and being a good friend to yourself. That way, you will respect your body and take better care of yourself. You will allow yourself to enjoy life, to love and be loved and to be happy because you no longer feel unworthy to experience these things, and your body image will no longer dictate the activities you can take part in. Changing your lifestyle out of self-love rather than self-hate is infinitely more rewarding.

MANAGING STRESS

Stress affects people in many different ways, and it can often lead to overeating (see page 90). If stress is causing you to overeat, try to identify its cause and find ways to eliminate it or, if that's not possible, develop strategies to alter your perception of it or your response to it.

Everyone reacts to and handles stress in his or her own way, but some coping strategies that might be helpful include learning to talk yourself through your stress response, relaxation techniques such as meditation or listening to relaxing music, and physical activity.

You can also seek guidance from professional counsellors or self-help books. If you are under stress at work, you should talk to your manager about it because employers now have a legal responsibility to resolve such problems when they are brought to their attention.

MANAGING YOUR TIME

One common cause of stress, and of bad eating habits such as skipping meals or relying on convenience foods, is a failure to manage your time effectively. Successful time management is about recognizing the difference between what is urgent and requires action right now, and what is important in the long run but requires no immediate action.

You may be familiar with Parkinson's Law – work expands to fill the time available. To avoid falling into this trap, consider reducing activities that are an inefficient use of your time and learn to say no to people when necessary. Delegate tasks where possible, both at home and at work, and resist the temptation to do everything yourself. Learning to trust in other people's ability by helping them to acquire certain skills can be empowering to both you and them. Think and plan ahead, and write a to-do list and stick to it so that you regain control of your time instead of letting your time be in control of you.

Approach major or unpleasant tasks by breaking them up into smaller, more manageable parts that can be tackled one at a time, and avoid procrastination. The stress created by putting off doing something that has to be done is often much greater than the stress of actually doing it. Once the decision is made to do something, the anxiety will fade.

GETTING SUPPORT

Changing your behaviour and lifestyle is infinitely harder, and may even prove unworkable, without the support or at least the cooperation of close family and friends. Occasionally, people around you may try to test your resolve with temptation or may even tease or mock you. They may have their own personal agenda for wanting to see you fail, or even be uneasy with the thought of you changing into someone more desirable, attractive or self-sufficient. In such situations, it may be wise to wait until you feel more confident before divulging your intentions, but sometimes actively enlisting people's help and support can win them over.

In the case of close family, changing your lifestyle will inevitably affect them so their support is extremely important. Explain your intentions and try to engage their active participation. You are infinitely more likely to make and maintain lifestyle changes when you have their consent and help.

Additional or alternative networks of support include commercial organizations such as slimming clubs. These have recently expanded their presence on the internet and their relative anonymity can make them an attractive alternative to face-to-face support groups. You might feel better able to ask for help or disclose personal experiences, struggles and feelings when you go online, but beware of sites that ask for money in return for 'guaranteed' weight loss.

UPDATING YOUR PERSPECTIVES

Here are some useful ways by which you can begin the process of updating your ideas.

Challenge false beliefs that can be disabling, such as:

- 'I can't do it.' Look at how other people managed it. What made them able to do it? What sacrifices did they have to make? Are you willing to make those same sacrifices?
- 'I don't have enough time.' Other people with similar responsibilities and commitments have been able to cope. You have to manage your time according to your priorities, and if they don't coincide with your goals, you have to lower your expectations.
- 'I have no willpower.' If you are reading this book then the will is surely there. What may be lacking is motivation. That is why it is so important to set realistic, manageable goals.
- 'I give up too easily.' This happens when you set over-ambitious goals, so set manageable ones and progress slowly rather than making drastic changes that may be painful.

Accentuate the positive:

- Focus on what you did right and not just one thing you may have done wrong.
- Be more positive and look for the good from situations, even from present and previous mistakes and failures, which you can use as a learning tool.
- Value yourself and your health. You need to make that a priority if you are to succeed.
- Believe that you can succeed. If you have good information about what has been shown to work, and you use that information sensibly, you can believe in what you are doing and be confident that it is going to work.

Eliminate the negative:

- Don't focus only on what you did wrong.
- Avoid jumping to conclusions. Not losing any weight one week doesn't mean the diet's not working. Perhaps you gained muscle tissue. Look at your overall weight trend.
- Don't generalize from just one experience. If you didn't like one exercise don't assume you won't enjoy any of them.
- Never allow past diet failures to cast doubts over your ability to lose weight in the future. They were based on information that you had then, which may have been poor.

FOOD CRAVINGS

Cravings for certain foods can become a form of psychological addiction that leads easily to overconsumption and weight gain. Chocolate is one of the most common foods involved, but it seems that any food with a high sugar or fat content can become addictive.

MARY came to the clinic because she was struggling in vain to lose the small amount of weight she had slowly gained over the past five years. She claimed to have a healthy lifestyle and even kept a food diary, which showed that she ate balanced meals throughout the day, including plenty of fresh fruits and vegetables. She also led a very active life, and either walked or cycled to work, depending on the weather. But eventually it emerged that there was, in fact, one small problem – chocolate. She was eating chocolate in one form or another every single day: milk, plain, with nuts, with raisins, white, organic … You name it, she was eating it. When challenged about her excessive intake, she was quite defensive at first but finally admitted that chocolate was probably the reason she couldn't lose weight. She just couldn't resist it, despite having tried over and over again to eat less of it.

WHAT CAUSES IT?

The concept of food addiction is a controversial one. The word 'addictive' describes any activity that is so pleasurable or rewarding that you need considerable willpower to resist repeating it. Few in the medical world would classify a desire for specific foods as a true addiction, because there appear to be no physical withdrawal symptoms when you abstain from them. However, many of the thought processes of people who admit to cravings for certain foods, most commonly chocolate, closely resemble those of a cocaine addict eager for another hit.

The desire for chocolate – which in women seems to be heightened at certain times during the monthly cycle – can sometimes be so intense that you may feel unable to control your behaviour. It is perhaps this, more than anything else, that may make you feel as if you have an addiction. However, research has revealed that, despite media claims, there is no one chemical or substance within chocolate that creates the cravings or pacifies the desire. The reward that is craved is the whole sensory experience that chocolate delivers: the taste, the aroma, and the melt-in-the-mouth texture from the fat combined with the sweetness from the sugar.

In fact, most of the foods that people claim to be addicted to are those that are highly palatable and high in fat or sugar, such as sweets, cakes and pastries. The addition of salt and spices to foods, which creates a savory taste, also increases palatability and so some people may develop an extreme desire for these foods. This explains the highly addictive nature of some fast foods that combine fat with sweet as well as savoury flavours.

The cause of this addictiveness lies in the way the brain works. Our brains have evolved to reward us with pleasurable sensations when we do things (such as eating or having sex) that benefit us and help ensure our survival as individuals and as a species. These pleasurable sensations are triggered by areas of the brain known as reward centres.

When its reward centres are stimulated, your brain releases pleasure-inducing substances called natural endorphins. These are your body's own intrinsic feel-good chemicals, closely related to morphine and responsible for the mild high you may have after eating certain foods. Your reward centres are designed to be activated by the moderate sweetness of natural foods, but the unnaturally high levels of sweetness in many manufactured foods can trigger unusually powerful responses from them. In the case of chocolate, other brain chemicals, resembling those found in cannabis, may also play a role. Unfortunately, this high is short-lived and cravings for another hit soon creep back. These cravings can also be triggered and intensified by visual images of chocolate, so marketing and advertising play a crucial role by acting as external stimuli.

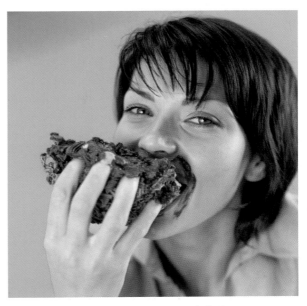

It's easy to eat more than you want, particularly if you eat it in hurry. Many people eat so quickly that their stomachs can't register fullness.

Other foods that can have an addictive quality include 'hot' foods – spicy chilli-based dishes such as fiery curries that create a sensation of heat. These foods trigger sensations that the body misinterprets as physical stress. This sets off an adrenaline rush that can also trigger the release of endorphins and so can become addictive, like high-adrenaline sports such as skydiving.

However, not all addictive behaviour is driven by desire. Sometimes it is driven by habits, some of which may have been instilled in you as a child. Just as many smokers refer to their addiction as a habit, so it can be with some foods. People often do things repeatedly out of habit and routine, even if it is to their detriment.

THE CONSEQUENCES

Hunger is an unpleasant sensation that acts as a strong incentive to eat, and so, in a sense, relieving hunger is like a reward in itself, and one that reinforces eating. The sensory appeal of food, however, has its own reward/reinforcement circuit in the brain. This is quite separate from – and more powerful than – the relief of hunger as a potential reward, and can make you want to eat, even when you're not hungry.

Manufactured foods are one of the main hazards facing people who are prone to food cravings. They combine highly concentrated sugars with fat, producing an intensely high taste sensation which, combined with the sight, aroma, and physical 'mouth-feel' of such foods, maximizes the stimulation of the brain's reward centres. The pleasure that follows then reinforces the urge to eat, regardless of when and how much you have eaten and dulling any feelings of fullness. The intense cravings you may feel when you try to abstain from such foods are not unlike the withdrawal symptoms that drug-addicted people experience, except they are psychological and not physical and serve to heighten your desire.

So the main difference between cravings for certain foods and normal hunger is that the desire to eat those foods comes purely from the pleasure that you expect from them. It is driven by pleasant memories of your previous experiences and not by a biological need to refuel.

THE CRAVING CYCLE

As for our case history, Mary (see page 128) was quietly proud of what she saw as her healthy lifestyle, and felt that it gave her the leeway to indulge in a little daily treat in the form of a bar of chocolate. Without giving it any real thought, she had convinced herself that this would have no effect on her health or weight and she didn't realize that her fondness for chocolate was a form of addictive behaviour.

As is the case with many addictive foods, chocolate is often seen as a guilty pleasure and an indulgence, which makes our relationship with it even more complex. Trying and failing to quit the chocolate-eating habit, as Mary had done repeatedly, can create a sense of powerlessness and loss of control. This can also mimic many of the feelings of drug-addicted individuals, and can even lead to cycles of bingeing and abstinence.

Unfortunately, the addictiveness of a food, and the extent to which it stimulates reward centres, tends to increase the more fat, refined carbohydrate and sugar it contains. Aside from the psychological consequences, eating such energy-dense foods – whether on a regular basis or by repeated episodes of bingeing – can increase your average daily calorie intake, and even if this is slight, it can lead to weight gain over time. If one kilo of fat represents 3500 calories, then even an extra 100 calories per day can theoretically make you gain 10 kilos in weight over the course of a year. And most average-sized chocolate bars contain up to 300 calories.

At first, Mary resisted the idea that she had an addiction to chocolate, but once she accepted it and realized that it was the cause of her weight gain, she was ready to begin a recovery programme that would help her to overcome her problem.

FOOD CRAVING RECOVERY PROGRAMME

1 FIND THE CAUSE

If you want to cure yourself of a constant desire for certain foods, you first need to check that your cravings are the result of an addiction and not symptoms of some other problem. For example, cravings may occur because your blood sugar is falling, either because you have not eaten enough or have been eating the wrong foods or as a form emotional hunger (see pages 94–9). The best way to exclude these is to keep a food diary (see page 120) to see if cravings are triggered by any emotionally stressful or uncomfortable situations and events.

You can also see if eating particular foods sets off the cravings. Do you get a taste for chocolate after you have eaten something that is artificially sweetened, like diet fruit yogurt? Does diet cola make you crave something savoury, such as crisps?

Remember that if cravings are not driven by a biological need or emotional hunger, then they are simply thoughts about food that can trigger your reward/reinforcement circuits, again, not dissimilar to the thoughts that a cocaine abuser may have about their last hit and which make them want another one.

2 AVOID EXTERNAL TRIGGERS

The smell from a bakery or the sight of confectionery at the supermarket checkout can set off cravings and so should be avoided where possible. Don't walk past the bakery on the way to work, and don't buy your newspaper at the corner shop where racks of sweets face you at the till. And don't browse the supermarket aisles – go prepared with a shopping list, go straight to the items that you need, and ignore the rest. Or, if you can, shop online and get your groceries delivered.

Other external triggers to beware of include activities that you associate with certain foods. For example, if going to the cinema makes you want popcorn, hot dogs, or ice cream, then you may have to make do with watching DVDs at home.

3 SET GOALS

Many people try to go 'cold turkey' and abstain suddenly and completely from their well-loved foods, but this often backfires. Behaviour, habits and tastes can take a long time to change, and if you try and you fail, you may end up feeling even more ashamed, disappointed, powerless and depressed. Food is different from other addictions because we all need it to live, whether we like it or not. It is not the same as alcohol, cigarettes or cocaine. Besides, you are constantly surrounded by food advertisements that tempt your palate. You must set small goals and make small changes only in the short term. Never say never again.

4 DELAY GRATIFICATION

The ability to look beyond immediate gratification towards the long term, and to learn to control your impulses, are important skills to develop. Keep reassuring yourself that you can kick the habit if you really want to, and remind yourself of the benefits that you will reap in the long run. If you still really want to eat the food that is causing problems, restrict yourself to a single small portion. The important thing is to remember the long-term goals you are hoping to achieve, and to compare the lasting pleasure you will experience later with the fleeting pleasure you are foregoing now.

PRACTICAL TIPS

• **Don't buy the foods that you find most addictive – if they are not to hand you are less likely to see them and want them. If you must keep them in the house, keep them out of sight.**

• **Don't deny yourself the food if you really want some, but at least try to buy smaller or even 'bite-size' portions and eat them sparingly. Add some salad or boiled or steamed vegetables to bulk up smaller-sized ready meals.**

• **Freeze chocolate; this makes it last longer in the mouth, so you can get a satisfying psychological reward with a smaller amount.**

• **Take your attention off your cravings by doing something distracting, such as phoning a friend, taking a relaxing bath or going for a walk.**

DIETARY GUIDELINES

If you want to lose weight, you have to reduce your overall total daily calorie intake. The healthiest and most natural way to do this is to eat foods that both help you to regulate your appetite and supply all the nutrients your body needs for good general health. Along with adopting a healthy diet you should increase the amount of exercise you take (see pages 140–49). This will help you to burn more calories, regulate your appetite, and improve your overall health while ensuring that you lose weight by shedding body fat and not muscle tissue.

These dietary guidelines are based on the current scientific knowledge about appetite, energy balance, nutrition and weight. The information they contain will help you to choose the kinds of foods likely to control your calorie intake and satisfy your appetite.

THE FOOD PYRAMID

'Food pyramids' (see page 50) are devices that illustrate the sorts of foods that you should eat more of and those that you should cut down on. They don't give exact proportions of the different kinds of food – for example by recommending that 50 percent of your daily intake should be vegetables and fruit – because that is neither helpful nor necessary. In addition, there is no definitive proof that rigid dietary structures based on precise numbers, percentages or ratios of different foods have any merit.

Some food pyramids also list the numbers of portions (servings) per day. Mine doesn't because it's intended only as a visual guide to changing the way that you eat: plenty of vegetables then decreasing amounts of lean protein, starchy carbohydrates and whole grains, legumes, low-fat dairy products, fruit, and small amounts of sweets, fats and oils.

Naturally, the types of food you actually eat will vary from meal to meal and from day to day, depending on the circumstances. Remember that what counts in the long run is what you do most of the time and not what you do some of the time.

In the long term, you will lose weight regardless of the ratios of fats, carbohydrates and protein in your food if there is a reduction in your overall daily calories. So it is actually possible to lose weight by increasing the amount of fat you eat while cutting down on carbohydrates and proteins. But in practice you should limit your intake of fat, because unlike high-fibre carbohydrate it provides no additional nutritional benefit, and unlike protein it has little effect on your appetite.

You can eat as much as you like of the right foods provided you become more aware of and pay attention to your intrinsic hunger cues: try to eat only when you are hungry, eat slowly, and stop eating when you feel comfortably full. When your diet is made up of healthy, nutritious foods that can regulate your appetite, you will

FOOD GROUPS AND DAILY SERVINGS*

FOOD GROUP	SERVINGS		TYPICAL SERVING SIZES
Bread, grains and cereals	4 to 9		one slice bread 25g (1oz) cereal 100g (3½oz) cooked grain, rice or pasta
Vegetables	5 to 7		75g (2¾oz) raw, leafy vegetables 40g (1½oz) non-leafy vegetables, cooked or raw 175ml (6fl oz) vegetable juice
Fruits	2 to 4		one medium-size fruit, such as an apple 125g (4½oz) chopped fresh, cooked or canned fruit 40g (1½oz) dried fruit 175ml (6fl oz) fruit juice
Meat, dried beans, nuts, eggs	2 to 3		85g (3oz) lean meat 85g (3oz) fish 85g (3oz) poultry 35g (1¼oz) nuts 2 tablespoons peanut butter 55g (2oz) cooked dried beans one egg
Dairy products	2 to 3		250ml (9fl oz) milk or yogurt 42g (1½oz) natural cheese 55g (2oz) processed cheese
Fats, oils and sweeteners	use sparingly		

- **Portion sizes** One of the simplest methods of measuring the right portion size is to use the size of your tightly closed fist as a guide. Your stomach is normally the size of a grapefruit, so the overall volume of food you eat at one meal – and which should trigger satiation – should be just slightly larger. This technique is especially useful when you are eating out.

find your calorie intake reduces automatically so these dietary guidelines do not specify any daily calorie limits. Calorie counting can make you obsessed with numbers, weights and measurements, and you will soon tire of it.

CARBOHYDRATES

Carbohydrates come in many different forms, but you should always choose quality carbohydrate foods that have nutritional value rather than just empty calories. These include high-fibre starchy carbohydrates, whole-grain cereals, legumes, fruit and vegetables. Try to avoid processed carbohydrates and foods containing refined sugars and sugar derivatives, including white flour and table sugar, and use the glycaemic index (see page 56) to find slow-release carbohydrates that provide sustained energy.

STARCHY CARBOHYDRATES AND WHOLE GRAINS

The term 'starchy carbohydrate' is loosely applied to whole grains and cereals such as wheat, oats, barley and rice, as well as bread, pasta and other products made from them. Root vegetables such as potatoes, sweet potatoes and yams are also generally classified as starchy carbohydrates. Barley, especially whole-grain 'pot' barley, has a very low GI compared to most other wholegrains and makes an ideal substitute for rice in many dishes.

The starchy carbohydrates and whole grains in your diet should be in as unrefined and natural a form as possible, with their fibrous bran layers or skins intact. This is because the quality of a refined carbohydrate tends to reduce with each step of processing — as a general rule, the finer they are ground into a powder, the higher their GI index.

LEGUMES

On the whole, it's a good idea to increase your intake of legumes (beans and pulses) because they tend to have low GIs, are high in fibre, contain a significant amount of protein and are of high nutritional value. Ideally, you should cook them from fresh, because canning increases their GIs. Soya beans and yellow split peas are the legumes with the lowest GI values.

VEGETABLES

Vegetables are, by and large, high-fibre slow-release carbohydrates with a high nutritional value and they should make up a big part of your daily food intake. Try to eat a wide range of vegetables with as much variety of colour and

HINTS AND TIPS FOR HEALTHY COOKING

As well as choosing the right foods, you should prepare and cook them carefully to retain their nutritional value and avoid adding extra calories.

- Instead of frying food in fat or oil, use cooking styles such as poaching, grilling, boiling, baking, roasting (without added fat) and steaming.
- If you want to fry, use one-calorie spray-on cooking oils or dry-fry with a non-stick pan.
- Before cooking, trim any visible fat from meat where possible and remove the skin from poultry.
- Vegetables should remain crunchy after cooking and pasta and whole grains should be al dente.
- Substitute soy sauce or fish sauce for oil when stir-frying.
- Use fruit purée (such as apple or prune) as a substitute for fat in baking.
- Substitute soya flour or whey protein powder for white flour in baking.
- Use chopped dried apricots or chopped prunes instead of raisins.
- Use fat-free fromage frais or yogurt as a base for dips, salad cream and sweet or savoury toppings.

HEALTHY FRUITS AND VEGETABLES

	Vitamin A*	Vitamin C	Vitamin E	Dietary fibre	Calcium	Iron	Folic acid
FRUIT							
Oranges		● ● ●		●			●
Grapefruit		● ● ●		●			●
Strawberries		● ● ●					●
Raspberries		● ● ●		● ●			●
Apricots:							
fresh	●	●			●	●	
canned	● ●	● ●			●	●	
dried	● ● ●	● ● ●		●	● ● ●	● ● ●	
Bananas		● ●		●			●
Papaya	● ● ●	● ● ●		●			
VEGETABLES							
Carrots	● ● ●	●		● ●			
Broccoli	● ● ●	● ● ●	●	●		●	● ●
Cabbage	● ●	● ●		●			●
Spinach	● ● ●	●	●	● ●		● ●	● ● ●
Peppers:							
red	● ● ●	● ● ●					
green	●	● ● ●					
Tomatoes	● ● ●	● ●	●				
Avocados	●		●	●			●

*As betacarotene

texture as possible, with plenty of bulky, fibrous vegetables such as broccoli, cauliflower, leeks and green beans because they are particularly good at making you feel full. Fresh vegetables are the best, but frozen vegetables are a good alternative and are preferable to canned, because freezing retains much more of the nutritional value than canning.

Include a mix of cooked, lightly cooked (crunchy) and raw vegetables in your diet because, although cooking destroys some of the fibrous structure and nutrients such as Vitamin C, it increases the availability of other nutrients, especially antioxidants. For example, the antioxidant lycopene becomes concentrated and is more readily absorbed from cooked tomatoes than from fresh. Lycopene is thought to help protect against certain diseases including heart disease and some forms of cancer, such as prostate cancer.

FRUIT

Most fruits are high in fructose (fruit sugar), which unlike glucose and other sugars is a slow-release carbohydrate. They are also high in natural fibre, most of which is in their skins, and like vegetables they have a high nutritional value. This is especially true of fruits with intensely coloured skins, including red apples and grapes, berries and black cherries, so eat the skins whenever possible.

Citrus fruits and fruits from temperate climates, such as apples, pears and plums, tend to have lower GIs and calorie contents than many that grow in warmer tropical climates, such as mangoes, pineapples and bananas. It is better to limit your consumption of such higher-calorie tropical fruits when trying to lose weight, but any fruit is better than none and infinitely better than sugary or high-fat snacks.

Ripening can increase the concentration of sugars in fruit, so ripe fruit tastes sweeter and has a higher GI than under-ripe fruit. Canning, drying and cooking fruit all increase its GI value and, as with vegetables, can destroy some nutrients while concentrating others, so aim for variety in the types of fruit you eat.

Fruit juice undeniably has some nutritional value, but weight for weight it is also considerably higher in calories than the fruit it is made from. Fruit juice also lacks fibre, which compromises its satiety value and may have adverse effects on your blood sugar levels, so try to drink it as part of a meal.

SWEETENERS

Refined sugars (such as table sugar) are extracted from plants such as sugar cane or sugar beet, and highly concentrated to produce a very sweet end-product that is devoid of fibre and lacking any nutritional benefit. They should be avoided.

Use alternative sweetening agents such as agave syrup, which has a very low GI value, or fruit juice concentrates. Honey and maple syrup are nutritionally superior to refined sugars, but they have high GIs and are relatively high in calories so should still be consumed in moderation. Sugar alcohols (polyols) also have lower GI values, but they are not widely available in shops and supermarkets.

Fructose, the sugar found naturally in most fruit, can also be manufactured and is available in bulk form in supermarkets. It has a much lower GI than other refined sugars, but recent studies have found that manufactured fructose can have harmful effects on blood fats so use it with caution.

LEAN PROTEIN

Proteins that contain all the essential amino acids are called complete proteins (see pages 58–9) and most from animal sources, including eggs and dairy products, fall into this category. Plant proteins, found in beans, nuts and seeds, are mostly incomplete.

Cuts of meat or poultry should be as lean as possible and any skin and visible fat should be removed prior to cooking. White meat from fish, seafood and poultry tends to be very lean and is preferable to the darker poultry meat, which is usually higher in fat. In general, you should try to buy and cook fresh or frozen meat and avoid pre-prepared meals that contain pastry, breadcrumbs or batter, or cream or curry sauces.

STARCHY CARBOHYDRATES

Avoid	Better	Best
Polished grains; fine polenta	Cracked wheat; coarse cornmeal; oatmeal; bran cereals; whole grain breakfast cereals	Whole grains (such as barley, rye, wheat); pure bran; whole oats
Sweet breakfast cereals		Whole-grain bread (such as pumpernickel)
White bread (all varieties)	Wholemeal pitta bread, tortillas; whole-grain crispbreads; matzos; oatcakes	Bran-fibre crispbreads
Melba toast; rice cakes; cream crackers	White pasta and basmati rice; brown rice	Whole-grain pasta
Rice noodles; fresh pasta	New potatoes; small baked potato	Brown basmati rice; wild rice
White rice; sweet rice		Sweet potatoes; yams
Mashed potato (including instant mash); roast potatoes; chips; crisps		

BEANS AND PULSES

Avoid	Better	Best
Canned in sauce, or with added sugar or salt	Canned in salt water (no added sugar)	Fresh or frozen

FRUIT

Avoid	Better	Best
Fruit canned in syrup	Fruit canned in fruit juice; fresh fruit juice	Fresh fruit, especially berries, citrus fruits and temperate climate fruits;
Dried fruit with added sugar	Dried fruit without added sugar	frozen berries; fresh fruit purée
Jam made with sugar; lemon curd; mincemeat	Jam made with pure fruit only	

PROTEINS

Avoid	Better	Best
Poultry skin, poussin; quail	Dark poultry meat (thighs, wings, drumsticks); duck; pheasant	White poultry meat; roast and minced poultry breast; rabbit
Kippers; fish roe; fishcakes	Mackerel; herring	White fish; seafood; salmon; smoked salmon; trout; tuna
Fish canned in oil	Fish canned in tomato sauce	Fish canned in brine or spring water
Standard mince beef, pork, lamb or poultry); burgers; sausages; kebabs; meat with visible fat; streaky bacon; crackling; ribs	Marbled meat	Lean meat; steak, cutlets or chops with no visible fat; minced beef or pork steak; lean roast beef slices
	Very lean beef or pork mince (half-fat)	
Turkey- or goose-liver pate; tongue (all varieties); pork kidneys	Chicken liver	Beef or lamb liver; heart (all varieties); beef, lamb or veal kidneys
Salami; frankfurters; chorizo; cured meats; deli meats; corned beef; pâté	Low-fat chicken or turkey roll; low-fat ham	Lean cooked ham
Egg yolks	Whole eggs	Egg whites
Tofu marinated in oil	Grilled tofu	Natural tofu

DAIRY PRODUCTS

Avoid	Better	Best
Full-fat cheese and milk	Half- or low-fat cheese	Low-fat cottage cheese
Extra-creamy, frozen and Greek yogurt; creme frâiche; cream; ice cream	Semi-skimmed milk	Skimmed milk
	Standard yogurt	Low-fat yogurt

FATS

Avoid	Better	Best
Coconut oil; palm oil; cooking or vegetable oil of unknown origin; modified oils; animal fats; shortening; suet; ghee; lard; dripping; goose fat; mayonnaise; margarines; trans-fats	Olive oil	Olives
	Avocado oil	Avocados
	Nut and seed oils	Nuts and seeds
	Linseed (flaxseed) oil	Linseeds (flaxseeds)
	Soya bean oil	Oily fish

DAIRY PRODUCTS

Low-fat cottage cheese or low-fat cream cheese are also good sources of protein. Low-fat yogurts contain some protein, but they can also contain added sugars so buy natural, unsweetened varieties and sweeten them with fruit or fruit purée.

FATS

A certain amount of fat is an essential part of a healthy diet, but most people in the West consume too much of it – standard dietary guidelines recommend that you get 30 percent of your daily calorie intake from fat, but this is still too much. For weight loss and long-term health, you need to reduce the amount of fat in your diet, especially the amount of saturated fat (see page 61). Switch to unsaturated fats from plant sources and oily fish wherever possible, and get them by eating whole nuts, seeds, olives and fish rather than from the purified oils obtained from them, because some of the nutrient content (including fibre and protein) is lost during extraction.

DRINKS

When you are dehydrated, you may begin to feel hungry so make sure you drink plenty of water or decaffeinated drinks. Have no more than three or four cups of tea or coffee per day because caffeine can be dehydrating. Green, white and herbal teas are better because they have lower levels of caffeine and are full of healthy antioxidants. Avoid adding milk to these teas because this will negate their benefits.

Red wine and fortified wines such as port have some benefits in the form of antioxidants. The current guidelines for sensible consumption of alcohol are: men 4 units and women 3 units per day.

THE BASIC PRINCIPLES OF A HEALTHY DIET

Follow these basic principles for a healthy diet that will lead to sustainable, long-term weight loss:

- Increase your consumption of fibrous, bulky whole-foods that require longer chewing times and induce satiation.
- Increase your intake of vegetables – aim for five portions (servings) per day.
- Eat unprocessed, high-fibre whole grains, beans and pulses that maintain satiety, stave off cravings and hunger and provide a steady flow of energy and nutrients to maintain your physical and mental stamina.
- Increase your intake of dietary fibre to at least 30 grams a day.
- Eat lean protein (especially fish) and low-fat dairy products that increase satiety.
- Eat fruit as a snack – aim for two portions a day, especially fruits with low GIs.
- Cut out all excess fat.
- Avoid processed or refined fast-release carbohydrates with high GIs – these lead to rapid changes in blood sugar levels associated with mood swings, cravings and fatigue.
- Avoid excess calories from foods and drinks that have no nutritional value.

EXERCISE GUIDELINES

Exercise, combined with dietary changes, is more likely to help you lose and maintain your weight than dietary changes alone. It promotes changes in your body that make you burn more calories – whether you are active or resting – and by influencing more subtle aspects of your body's energy regulation, such as appetite and mood, it helps you to adhere to your weight loss programme.

Physical activity is particularly important in the prevention of obesity, especially during childhood and adolescence, and the amount of exercise you take is an important predictor of your future health. Rates of both mortality (death) and morbidity (illness) are lower among people who take plenty of exercise, as are the incidences of heart disease, cancer and mental problem such as depression. Exercise has been shown to improve blood pressure, stabilize blood sugar levels, and reduce the amount of harmful fats in the blood while boosting the levels of healthy ones. So there are many good reasons for taking exercise – it's more than just a useful aid to weight loss.

WHAT TYPE OF EXERCISE?

The type and amount of extra exercise you will need to help you lose weight will depend to a degree on your goals and how active you already are. If you rate yourself as highly inactive, then begin by reducing the time you spend in sedentary pursuits such as watching TV, especially during the daytime. For example, if you tend to rely on someone else to do most of the household chores, such as ironing, cleaning and preparing meals, start burning more calories by doing more of them yourself.

Thereafter, increase coincidental or opportunistic activity if you have a busy schedule and lack leisure time, for instance by walking to the shops, work or school instead of taking the car, getting off the bus one stop earlier and walking the rest of the way, and always using the stairs instead of the lift. Alternatively, or in addition to opportunistic activity, take part in more leisure-time activities and sports, such as dancing, tennis, bowling, swimming or outdoor pursuits like hill-walking, rambling and cycling that get you out and about. The most important thing is to choose one or several activities that you enjoy.

MAKE SURE YOU'RE FIT FOR EXERCISE

If it's a while since you took any regular exercise, get your doctor to give you a thorough physical examination before undertaking anything strenuous.

If you want a more structured exercise programme, then ideally it should include some cardiovascular (aerobic) exercise to condition your heart, lungs and circulation and improve your stamina, and resistance training (a form of anaerobic exercise) to increase your muscle mass and strength (see pages 37–9). Both these forms of exercise will help you to lose fat, and you should combine them with stretching exercises to reduce muscle tension, increase flexibility and help prevent injuries. These exercises can be carried out in a gym or at home, whichever you prefer.

HOW MUCH TO DO

Cardiovascular exercise of moderate intensity is any activity that involves the use of large muscle groups (such as those in your arms or legs) to move a heavy load, including your body weight. This type of exercise includes brisk walking or slow jogging, cycling, swimming or rowing, and using gym equipment such as an exercise cycle or a rowing machine. Start gently at a pace that reflects your age, current fitness and mobility, and slowly build up to a comfortable yet challenging intensity – one at which you can still hold a conversation while you are exercising. The Borg Scale (page 143) and The Talk Test (page 144) will help you to judge the intensity of the exercise you are taking.

When you exercise, you should focus on the total amount of physical stress, effort and fatigue involved and not on any one factor such as leg pain or shortness of breath. Aim for moderate intensity exercise (5 or 6 on the scale); a rating of 8 or above is too hard. What you should not focus on is the number of calories you are burning, as this is highly variable between individuals and is not the overall purpose of the exercise.

You can also use your heart rate to assess how hard you are exercising. If your THR is towards the lower end of

YOU CAN'T CHOOSE WHERE YOU LOSE IT

Neither resistance training nor aerobic exercise can spot-reduce body fat. Where the body loses fat from is largely determined by your gender, age, hormonal status and genetic inheritance and cannot be altered by exercise alone. What exercise can do, however, is to develop the muscles beneath the layers of fat, reducing a flabby appearance and giving greater definition to the shape of the muscles.

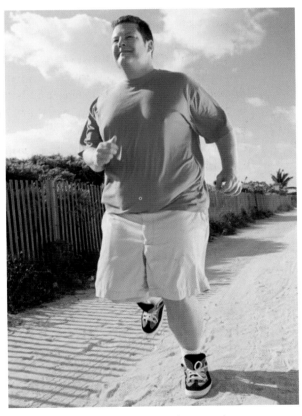

Exercise combined with a weight-loss diet not only will help you lose weight faster but will make you look much better.

FINDING YOUR TARGET HEART RATE

This table shows the average target heart rate ranges for people of different ages. You can measure your heart rate during an exercise session by taking your own pulse – count the number of pulses in a 15-second period, and multiply that by 4 to get your heart rate in beats per minute. Alternatively you could use a heart-rate monitor, which will measure your heart rate continuously while you are exercising.

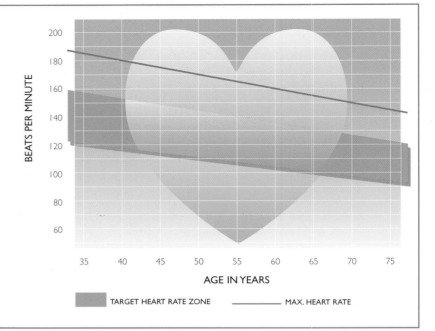

the range for your age when you are exercising, then you are not working hard enough, but if it is near the upper end then you are exercising too hard and should ease off.

Exercise for short lengths of time, even for as little as five minutes to begin with, and increase gradually to a target of thirty to forty minutes per day, ideally every day but at least five days a week. The total exercise time can be split into say, ten- or fifteen-minute sessions if that is more convenient or manageable. Bear in mind that endorphins and adrenaline levels increase after about 20 minutes and peak after about 40 minutes and it takes approximately 20 minutes for your body to access its fat stores, so aim to do at least 20 minutes of continuous activity whenever possible.

Resistance training that involves lifting weights can be interspersed with cardiovascular exercise or performed on its own. When you do resistance training (also called strength training), target specific muscle groups such as your upper body, back or legs on separate days so that they get enough time to recover, which is as important for muscle growth as the exercise itself. Too often people over-exercise, and this is definitely one instance where less is more.

Resistance training relies as much on technique as intensity to achieve results, and there are numerous variations on each exercise, but it can lead to injury if you do it incorrectly. It is, therefore, advisable to get proper instruction from a well-qualified professional, even if only for one session – especially if you are a beginner. You can do the exercises at home using household items such as cans and bottled water as weights, so at the very least, a book or video that illustrates the exercises clearly is a must. Start with light weights or resistance and increase the intensity gradually to minimize the risk of injury.

Whenever you do cardiovascular or resistance training, you should end the session with stretching exercises. Again, proper instruction on correct stretching is vital because poor technique can cause injury. If you want to do stretching exercises at any other time, never do them with 'cold' muscles – do some warming-up exercises first.

EQUIPMENT

Most forms of exercise involve using some sort of equipment, and it's worth investing in well-made, good-quality kit that will be reliable and safe to use. For example, walking – the easiest, cheapest and one of the best forms of exercise – will be more enjoyable if you wear a comfortable pair of quality sports shoes. And if you buy a pedometer, a device that counts the steps you take, you can monitor your daily walking activity and set yourself targets to aim for. For cardiovascular exercise and resistance training, there is a wide range of machines and equipment available to buy or rent for home use, covering every budget and taste, along with numerous exercise instruction books, DVDs and videos.

Before you make any big investment in exercise equipment, though, think it

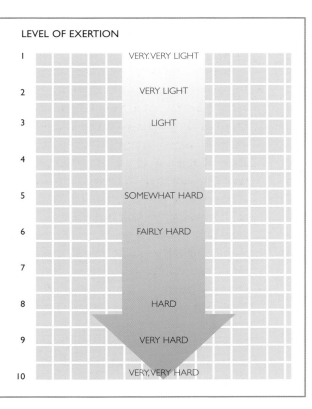

HOW TO USE THE BORG SCALE

The Borg Rating of Perceived Exertion (RPE) Scale, devised in the late 1950s by Swedish exercise physiologist Gunnar Borg, is an easy way to assess how hard your body is working during exercise. There are a number of different versions of the Borg Scale, but the most common are this simple 1–10 scale and one that runs from 6 to 20, in which the '6' represents a heart rate of 60 beats per minute and the '20' a heart rate of 200.

To use this scale, estimate how much exertion you are putting into your exercise – for instance light or somewhat hard – and see where that falls on the scale. In general, you should aim to exercise at a level of about 5 or 6, and avoid reaching a level of 8 or above.

LEVEL OF EXERTION

1	VERY, VERY LIGHT
2	VERY LIGHT
3	LIGHT
4	
5	SOMEWHAT HARD
6	FAIRLY HARD
7	
8	HARD
9	VERY HARD
10	VERY, VERY HARD

CAN YOU PASS THE TALK TEST?

A very easy way to judge the intensity of the exercise you are taking is to use the Talk Test.

If you are moving and ...

- your breathing increases but you can carry on a conversation
- you feel a little warm
- you break a light sweat

... then it is just right.

through carefully to be sure that it offers the kind of exercise that really appeals to you and is likely to become a long-term part of your lifestyle. The same applies to gym memberships, which are expensive but so often wasted. Ask for trial sessions before signing up, to ensure that working out in a gym is something you really want to do. Take into account the location of the gym and its accessibility at the times of day you are planning to go there – will it still appeal

HOW SUPPLE ARE YOU?

Before starting regular stretching exercises, it helps to know how supple you are now. One way to do this is the 'sit and reach test', which involves attempting to touch your toes from a seated position. To do this test, sit with your feet together and your legs out straight in front of you. Point your toes towards the ceiling. Bending from the waist and keeping your legs on the floor, stretch your arms forward to reach your toes. An average or below-average result indicates that you should concentrate on improving your suppleness. A good result indicates that, while suppleness is not a major problem for you, you should still include flexibility exercises in your fitness programme to maintain your current level.

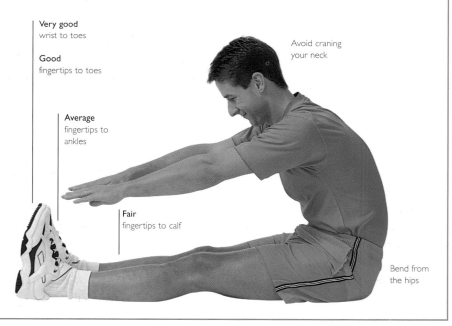

Very good
wrist to toes

Good
fingertips to toes

Average
fingertips to ankles

Fair
fingertips to calf

Avoid craning your neck

Bend from the hips

HOW STRONG ARE YOU?

The abdominal curl test is a good way to help you determine your current level of muscular ability. To do an abdominal curl, lie on your back with your shoulders resting on the floor, arms by your sides. Lift your head and shoulders off the floor so that your hands slide forward 10 cm (4 in) and then carefully lower your head and shoulders again. Breathe out as you curl up and breathe in as you lower back down. Do as many as you can in one minute and compare the result with the ratings chart shown below.

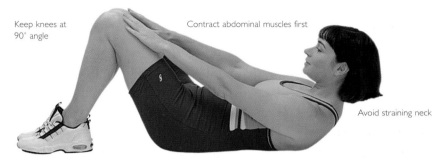

Keep knees at 90° angle

Contract abdominal muscles first

Avoid straining neck

Keep lower back in contact with the floor

WOMEN

Age	Very fit	Fit	Average	Unfit
40–50	35+	31–35	24–30	below 23
51–60	30+	26–30	20–25	below 19
60+	25+	21–25	15–20	below 14

MEN

Age	Very fit	Fit	Average	Unfit
40–50	39+	35–39	29–34	below 29
51–60	34+	30–34	24–29	below 24
60+	29+	25–29	19–24	below 19

on a cold, dark, midwinter night on your way back from a hard day at work? Will using the gym fit around other commitments that cannot be changed? Are you confident about exercising with other people, or would you be happier exercising alone at home? These are all points worth considering before committing yourself to membership.

Finally, remember that we each have our own individual capacity for exercise and its results are not immediate. If you see working out as a chore rather than a valuable part of your lifestyle, you are more likely to abandon exercise out of disappointment, dislike or boredom.

Suggested Exercises

Any exercise programme should include different types of exercise. The most important to include are ones for stamina, muscle toning and stretching. As your stamina improves, you can increase the time spent on each exercise. A beginning programme should last at least 20 minutes and you should work up to 40 minutes to achieve optimum fitness benefits.

Always do a warm-up routine before you start and a cool-down at the end to reduce the risk of injury and aches and pains. After you finish, a breathing exercise may be relaxing.

FOR STAMINA
LEG AND ARM CURLS

1 Stand tall with your shoulders upright and facing forwards and your feet hip-width apart. Keep your elbows at your sides, your hands low in front of you and fists slightly clenched.

2 Raise your hands to your shoulders. At the same time, lift your right heel up to your buttocks, transferring your weight. Lower your hands as you lower your foot to the floor. Repeat with the other foot. Do this at a steady, even pace. Continue for up to 2–3 minutes.

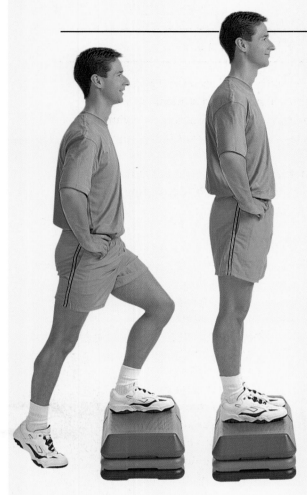

STEP-UPS

Step on and off a sturdy box 10–20 cm (4–8 in) high (or a step) for up to 3 minutes. First, step up with the left foot, then the right, and then step down with the right foot, followed by the left. Fully straighten the knees each time you step up, but don't lock them. Keep an even, regular pace – up, up, down, down. Continue for up to 3 minutes.

STAR JUMPS

1 Stand tall with your feet slightly apart and your arms by your sides. Bend your knees and then spring upwards, raising both arms above your head at the same time. Land with your feet well apart and knees in line with your toes.

2 Now, spring upwards and land with your feet together and your arms at your sides. Repeat for up to 30 seconds.

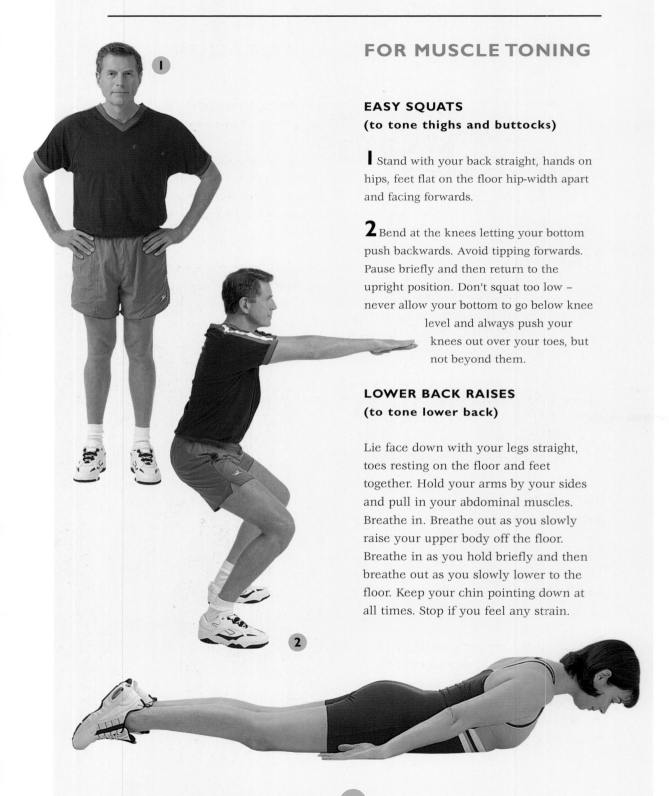

FOR MUSCLE TONING

EASY SQUATS
(to tone thighs and buttocks)

1 Stand with your back straight, hands on hips, feet flat on the floor hip-width apart and facing forwards.

2 Bend at the knees letting your bottom push backwards. Avoid tipping forwards. Pause briefly and then return to the upright position. Don't squat too low – never allow your bottom to go below knee level and always push your knees out over your toes, but not beyond them.

LOWER BACK RAISES
(to tone lower back)

Lie face down with your legs straight, toes resting on the floor and feet together. Hold your arms by your sides and pull in your abdominal muscles. Breathe in. Breathe out as you slowly raise your upper body off the floor. Breathe in as you hold briefly and then breathe out as you slowly lower to the floor. Keep your chin pointing down at all times. Stop if you feel any strain.

STRETCHES

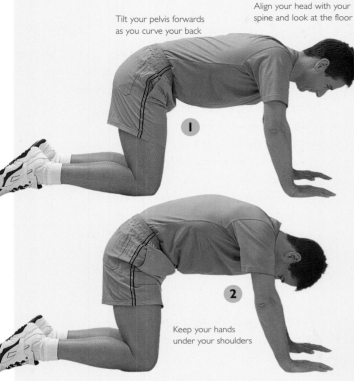

Tilt your pelvis forwards as you curve your back

Align your head with your spine and look at the floor

Keep your hands under your shoulders

BACK STRETCH
(for the lower spine)

I Get on your hands and knees on the floor, hands under shoulders, fingers pointing forwards and knees hip-width apart.

2 Pull your abdomen up towards your spine and curve your back. Hold for up to 10 seconds and then relax your back.

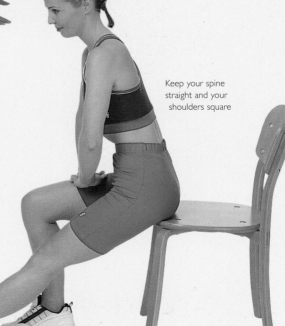

Keep your spine straight and your shoulders square

BACK OF THIGHS
(for the upper legs)

I Sitting on the edge of a chair, place one foot flat on the floor. Extend the other leg in front of you, with your heel on the floor.

2 Placing your hands on your thigh, lean forwards from the hips and feel the stretch in the back of the thigh on the straight leg. Repeat on the other side.

SHOPPING GUIDELINES

In the past, it was easy to work out which foods were low in calories and which were laden with sugar and fat, and because people prepared and cooked their food using fresh ingredients, they could decide the fat and sugar content of their meals. If you wanted to control your weight, you made foods such as fresh fruit and vegetables, lean meat and fish the basis of your diet, and ate obviously fattening foods such as dairy products, sweets and cakes in moderation.

These basic principles still apply today, but most of us lead busy lives that discourage us from buying, preparing and cooking food from fresh ingredients. We just don't have the time, so we opt for manufactured foods that we can simply heat and eat. These are tasty and convenient, but unless you choose them wisely they can be a major source of excess calories in your diet.

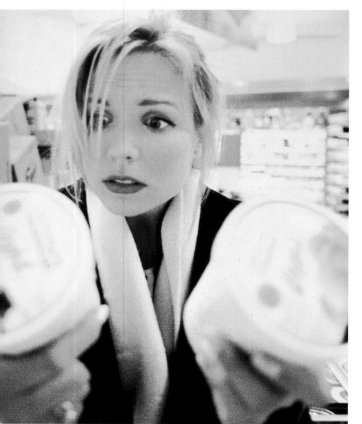

Today, you almost feel as though you need an degree in label reading in order to determine what exactly is in your food. Manufacturers often use confusing chemical names.

HIDDEN FATTENERS

When shops and supermarkets started selling pre-prepared convenience foods, our eating habits began to change dramatically. Since then, we have all become increasingly reliant on foods that have been entirely or partially prepared or cooked for us by their manufacturers. Whether these manufactured foods are entire meals including side orders, or sweet or savoury snacks such as confectionery bars, biscuits and crisps, or any number of beverages, almost all of us rely on them to some extent. This reliance is why it is vital to have a good understanding of the nutritional and calorific value of such foods if you want to gain greater control over what and how much you are eating.

For example, many manufactured foods contain substantial quantities of hidden fat or sugar in addition to the amounts that we can clearly see and taste. We know from experience that some foods are likely to be high in such

AVOIDING SOME
COMMON PITFALLS

When you become familiar with food labels and more confident in interpreting their data, you will be able to compare different foods so that you can make healthier choices when shopping. The information on the labels can help you to avoid those hidden and/or harmful fats, refined sugars and carbohydrates that are sometimes lurking unexpectedly in some unlikely products.

- Always check the calorie count of foods labelled 'sugar-free' or 'fat-free', because those terms don't mean 'calorie-free'. These foods often contain virtually the same number of calories as the standard varieties.

- Never assume anything about the calorie count of a convenience meal or other manufactured product that's a version of a food we traditionally think of as being low in calories. Always check the calorie content.

- Manufacturers can make a lower-calorie version of a product either by adding water, air or other 'fillers' to make it less calorie-dense, or by making the portion size smaller. The product may be crispier, more porous, or runnier, but remains essentially unchanged.

- Always check the portion size, because that specified by the manufacturer may not always be the amount that you are likely to eat at any one time or would feel satisfied with. Don't be misled by what appears, on first sight, to be a very small calorie count per serving.

ingredients. Sweet foods such as cakes, biscuits and confectionery, and savoury foods such as crisps, pies and pastries, obviously fall into this category and it is easy to eliminate such sources of fat and sugar from our diets.

But some foods are more ambiguous and made even more so by their labelling. Fat-free frozen yogurt sounds like it should be healthy and low in calories, but is it really? Sugar-free or low-fat biscuits seem likely to be lower in calories than their standard counterparts and therefore a better choice, but are they? When you look at a supermarket shelf stocked with ten different tomato-based cooking sauces, how can you tell which is likely to be the best choice? Many convenience foods contain a surprising amount of hidden unhealthy and modified fats and sugars despite outward appearances, and some that are promoted as healthy or 'good for you' turn out to be no better than others.

The only way to identify genuinely healthy manufactured foods that are likely to help you lose weight is to gain greater familiarity with their ingredients and their nutritional content. Failing that, you will have to rely on the judgement and honesty of the food manufacturers, and even though some are reliable, remember that ultimately their aim is to provide products that people like and at prices that they are willing to pay. Their responsibility does not extend to the health of the nation. It is important that we as individuals take some responsibility for our own food choices and learn for ourselves how to get the best from what is available.

FOOD LABELLING

All pre-packaged foods must, by law, be labelled with a list of their ingredients. In addition, food manufacturers often provide additional data about the macronutrient, and sometimes even micronutrient, content of their products. However, some also use all sorts of clever (but legal) techniques to disguise the true nature of the ingredients, and mislead consumers with bold, eye-catching claims about the merits of their products. You have to look beyond the hype and learn how to interpret ingredient lists and nutritional labelling. By knowing what to look out for and what to avoid, you can avoid those hidden fats and sugars that may be sabotaging your attempts to lose weight (see Appendix, page 156).

THE INGREDIENTS LIST

The ingredients lists on many manufactured food products are becoming so detailed that many people find them hard to understand. The packaging of a standard loaf of bread, for example, can list over ten ingredients, that of a simple cooking sauce over twenty, and those of products such as cakes well over thirty different ingredients, depending on the variety. Even so, these lists are modest compared to those of specialist foods such as sports nutrition bars, which can contain over fifty ingredients. Many foods also contain additives that act as preservatives, colouring and sweetening agents, thickeners, emulsifiers, bulking agents and humectants (moisture retainers) that improve the products' shelf-life and sensory appeal.

The ingredients of a food product are listed in descending order of weight, measured at the 'mixing bowl stage' when the food was being prepared. The major components appear at the beginning of the ingredients list and those appearing towards the end are present in smaller and smaller quantities. Where the list is very long, the main contributors to the overall calorific value of the food are

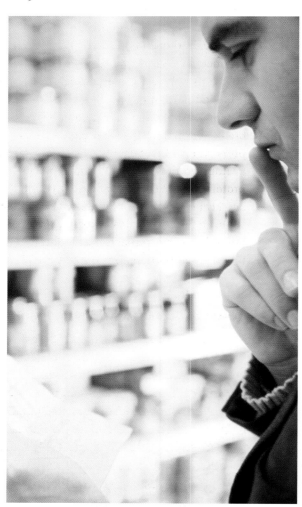

The plethora of products on supermarket shelves can mean lots of time poring over labels to check which particular item is the healthiest.

therefore likely to be among the first seven or so ingredients. Thereafter, the ingredients tend to make a less significant contribution to calorie content.

NUTRITIONAL DATA

The ingredients list, although useful, often doesn't give you all the information you need about a product. It won't tell you, for example, how energy-dense it is. This is important because the ingredient list for a food may show that it contains fat and sugar, but usually it won't tell you how much. You can guess at this from the order in which they appear in the list, but you won't know whether they are present in large quantities or in amounts too small to make a significant contribution to the calorie content. This is why you need to be able to read and interpret nutritional data.

The nutritional data (or nutrition facts) on food packaging is information that tells you the amounts of fat, carbohydrate, protein, calories and occasionally fibre that a product contains. In the United Kingdom and other European countries, nutritional data is usually given per package of a product or for 100 grams of it, and for a specified portion of it.

For example, the information below is taken from the label on a packet of breakfast cereal. This label gives extensive nutritional data, including the types and proportions of dietary fibre as well as fats and carbohydrates, for 100 grams and for an average portion. Each 100 grams of this cereal contains 2.7 grams of fat, 11.2 grams of protein and 67.6 grams of carbohydrate. It has a fair amount of dietary fibre, but at 340 kcal (dietary calories) per 100 grams, it is still a calorie-dense food.

In the United States, nutritional data is given for specified portions only. This is helpful in some respects, but it doesn't allow you to compare different foods directly because the portion sizes quoted vary from one product to another. Another feature of

NUTRITIONAL DATA ON A TYPICAL PACKET OF BREAKFAST CEREAL

	Per 37.5g	Per 100g
Energy	540 kj/128 kcal	1440 kj/340 kcal
Protein	4.2g	11.2g
Carbohydrate	25.4g	67.6g
(of which sugars)	(1.8g)	(4.7g)
Fat	1.0g	2.7g
(of which saturates)	(0.2g)	(0.6g)
Fibre	3.9g	10.5g
(of which soluble)	(1.2g)	(3.2g)
(of which insoluble)	(2.7g)	(7.3g)
Sodium	0.1g	0.27g

US food labelling is the percentage daily value (%DV) given for each of the important dietary constituents of a product. These are calculated from the Dietary Guidelines for Americans, published every five years by the US Department of Health and Human Services and the Department of Agriculture. The percentage daily values are based on the nutritional needs of an average adult who consumes 2000 calories a day.

The nutritional information, see right, shows how the percentage daily values are given on typical US food labels, in this case the label of a savoury sauce. For an average-weight person who is moderately active and consumes 2000 calories a day, one 40-gram serving of this particular product will provide 36 percent of the daily recommended fibre intake, 34 percent of the recommended protein intake and 6 percent of the recommended daily fat intake.

NUTRITION FACTS
(FROM A SAUCE LABEL)

Serving size 40g
Servings per container 9
Calories 150
Calories from fat 35

Amount per serving	%DV
Total fat 4g	6%
Sat fat 1g	5%
Cholesterol 0g	0%
Sodium 210 mg	9%
Potassium 30 mg	1%
Total carbs 12g	4%
Fibre 9g	36%
Sugars 0g	0%
Protein 17g	34%

SMALL CUTS MAKE A DIFFERENCE

Looking at nutrition labels and choosing the foods that contain fewer calories than their rival products may seem trivial, especially when the differences in calorie content are not that large. But remember that although no one product can help you to lose weight, cutting calories across a range of the foods that you eat each day can, over a period of time, add up to a significant reduction in your overall calorie intake. For example, changing the foods you eat so that you cut just 20 calories from your breakfast cereal, 20 from your lunch, 10 from snack biscuits, 30 from your dinner and 20 from your dessert adds up to 100 fewer calories in a day. If you kept that up for six months you would reduce your total energy intake over that period by more than 18,000 calories, which equates to a weight loss of more than 5 kg.

QUICK-REFERENCE SYSTEM

If you want to use nutritional data to assess the health values of foods and make comparisons between different products, it's a good idea to develop a quick-reference system based on reading the ingredients list, the calorie count, then the fat, sugar and fibre content.

- Check the ingredients list to get a quick idea of the likely amounts of processed carbohydrates, refined sugars and fat that a product contains. If any are listed towards the beginning, then the product may contain high levels of them.

- Look at the calorie content of the food and roughly calculate the amount that 100 grams would contain, if that is not the amount quoted. Any food that contains more than about 300 calories per 100 grams is an energy-dense food, and you will need to control the portion size carefully if you want to keep your calorie intake down.

- Look at the fat content. Foods that contain more than 5 or 6 grams of fat per 100 grams, even when the fat is derived from a healthy natural source such as nuts, are likely to be calorie-dense and so again should be eaten in moderation. Excess consumption of foods containing high amounts of fat may make weight control harder to achieve.

- Check the carbohydrate content of the food, and in particular the proportions of sugars. If the product is made mainly of fruit, then a high sugar content may reflect the presence of natural sugars derived from the fruit. But if the product also lists some form of added sugar among the ingredients, then it becomes much harder to identify the relative proportions of refined and natural sugars. In general, if 100 grams of a product contains more than about 30 grams of sugars, whether natural or refined, then it is a high-sugar, energy-dense food and should be eaten in small portions only.

- Finally, check the fibre contents when comparing breads, breakfast cereals and other foods consisting mainly of carbohydrates. Ideally, such products should be made of whole grains and contain as much fibre as possible. Products such as wholemeal bread or pasta should contain at least 7 grams of total fibre per 100 grams, and cereals based on wheat bran and oat bran contain as much as 15 to 20 grams of fibre per 100 grams and so are excellent choices.

APPENDIX: CHECK THE LABEL

CARBOHYDRATES

When you are trying to lose weight, there are two types of carbohydrate to avoid: refined starches and refined sugars, from which most or all of the valuable dietary fibre has been removed. These processed and concentrated carbohydrates are now found in a large number of chilled, frozen and canned convenience foods and snacks. Unfortunately, manufacturers use a variety of different terms for them in the ingredients lists (usually chemical names unfamiliar to the average consumer) in an attempt to disguise their presence.

STARCHES

Refined starches are essentially complex carbohydrates derived mainly from cereal grains, rice, potatoes and occasionally from legumes such as soya beans and chickpeas. The process of refining and milling usually involves the removal of the fibre, leaving just the available starch element of the original carbohydrate. This starch is sometimes chemically altered to produce what are called 'modified' starches.

Refined starches are found in a wide variety of items, from baked goods to pasta and polenta, in breadcrumbs and batter to coat meat, as fillers in sausages and burgers and as thickening agents in yogurts and sauces. Small amounts are inconsequential, but where possible they should be avoided.

When buying foods made from or containing flour, choose the whole grain varieties – this should be clearly stated in the ingredients list. If the ingredients do not specify whole, whole grain or whole meal, then assume that the fibre has been removed. The term 'bran' on the ingredients list also indicates fibre, which may be derived from different sources including wheat, oats, rice and soya.

Gram flour (made from chickpeas) and soya flour have a higher protein and fat content than cereal grain flour and rice flour, and because they often retain much of the fibre they have a lower GI.

SUGARS AND SWEETENERS

Sugars are very common in packaged and processed foods, and make a big contribution to their calorie counts. Sometimes the label lists them simply as sugar, but they are less obvious when listed by their chemical names, which include sucrose, glucose, dextrose and fructose. Sugars represent empty calories and have no nutritional value.

Many food items labelled 'sugar free' or 'no added sugar' are sweetened using a variety of different agents in place of highly refined sugars. These agents may include fruit juice, agave syrup, maple syrup, honey, sugar alcohols and artificial sweeteners. Fruit juices are usually clearly stated and their source is often given. These, together with agave syrup, tend to have relatively low GIs, so they are better alternatives to refined sugar. They also have some nutritional value, so they provide more than just empty calories. However, all these agents will add to your daily calorie intake, so consume them in moderation.

Sugar alcohols or polyols, such as mannitol, sorbitol, and erythritol, are more slowly metabolized than refined sugars, so they don't affect blood sugar levels in the same way. Furthermore, weight for weight they have a much lower calorific content.

Artificial sweeteners such as sucralose are described as 'non nutritive', a term used to imply that they have no calorific or energy content. Their use is now widespread, (even in foods not labelled 'sugar free'), either alone or in combination with other sweetening agents such as polyols or with refined sugar. Weight for weight, they have sweetening strengths that are hundreds of times greater than that of refined sugar. Their safety and use in foods is controversial, although they appear to have a good safety record if consumed in moderate quantities.

GLYCERINE

Glycerine (also called glycerin or glycerol) is a carbohydrate used in manufactured foods, such as cereal bars and nutrition bars, as both a humectant and a sweetening agent. Gylcerine contains calories but is metabolized slowly and so won't significantly affect blood sugar levels.

PROTEIN

On the whole, protein is not an ingredient to be avoided in convenience foods, because it is an essential part of a healthy diet, generally has a low GI and can add bulk to food. The ingredients list generally states the source of any protein it contains if it is derived from meat, for example, chicken, beef or pork protein. On meat and meat products, it will also state the percentage of the food that is made up of meat – for example, roast chicken may contain 97 percent chicken, plus sugar and salt. When looking at meat and meat product labels, it's a good idea to check the exact amount of meat or protein as some products contain smaller amounts than expected. For instance, chicken nuggets may contain only 70 percent chicken, the remainder being added water, carbohydrate fillers, flavourings and the batter coating. If the amount of meat in a food that is primarily a protein source is stated as less than 85 percent, it should be avoided as this would tend to suggest that the product contains added fat, refined carbohydrates or additives.

As well as using meat or other protein-rich foods as ingredients in their products, manufacturers also use proteins isolated from various sources to increase protein content or to provide texture or bulk. These protein isolates include soya, whey, dairy, vegetable and pea proteins, calcium caseinate and mycoprotein. Protein isolates are also sold as food supplements, and can be a useful way of supplementing protein intake, especially for vegetarians.

FAT

The presence of fat is quite easy to spot in ingredients lists. Essentially, any term including the words 'oil' or 'fat' refers to a dietary fat. What may be harder to ascertain is the amount and type of fat and its contribution to the overall calorific value of a particular food. This information is generally only available in the nutritional data (see page 153).

INDEX

ACKNOWLEDGEMENTS

Carroll and Brown Publishers would like to thank:

Production Director Karol Davies
Computer Management Paul Stradling
Picture Researcher Sandra Schneider
Proofreader Geoffrey West

Picture credits
Getty Images
Front cover, page 2, page 4 (bottom), page 12,
page 18, page 22, page 24, page 42, page 77,
page 79, page 81, page 97, page 100, page 108,
page 121, page 123, page 150, page 152
page 68 (Foodpix)
page 70, page 116, page 119, page 141 (Altrendo)